MY GOD, MY GOD!

MY GOD, MY GOD!

Answers to Our Anguished Cries

By

Ruth Vaughn

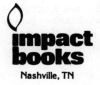

impact
books

Nashville, TN

First Printing March 1982.

14023p

Library of Congress Cataloging in Publication Data
Vaughn, Ruth.
    My God, my god!
    1. Vaughn, Ruth. 2. Christian biography—United States. 3. Endocrine glands—Diseases—Patients—United States—Biography. I. Title.
BR1725.V36A35   209'.2'4 [B]   81-84925
ISBN 0-86608-006-6   AACR2

Distributed by The Zondervan Corporation.

Cover design by Rip Carloss
Interior design by Nancye Willis

Contents

Foreword

In my mail today I found the completed manuscript of this book, and a long letter from a dear friend whom I have never seen—Ruth Vaughn. The letter, as I have come to expect from Ruth, was beautiful. It was filled with amazing insights. It was honest. And it was even more stimulating than usual—and *that* is saying a *lot!*

Quite frankly, I had planned to begin a new book manuscript of my own today. God had better plans.

I read Ruth's letter and it sent me straight to her manuscript. Not that she was pressing me for a reaction; I went because I simply could not resist.

Of course, I meant only to read a few pages. It is now late afternoon. I have just finished the entire book. I did not arise from the chair until I had read every word through tears. Her open, honest, perceptive sharing, beautifully written, teaches *me* about my own beliefs in God's eagerness to redeem everything.

In her letter, Ruth wrote: "As you have been a part of my life, so you are a part of this sharing. As I have agonized over the opening of this personal record, an acute point of pain has been that you might be embarrassed to be a part of it . . . For, dearest Genie, it *is* your philosophy *at work* in the debris of my life plans."

Over the years I have read hundreds of pages of Ruth Vaughn's writings. Only in the above quotation from today's letter have I ever found a really poor, inadequate, distorted use of a word: *embarrassed!*

Embarrassed!

I have never been so *honored* in my life—and although I use this word almost not at all in my vocabulary—I have never been so *humbled.*

For years, Ruth has written to me and kept me attempting to communicate my Christian beliefs by assuring me that one blazing insight God gave me has, in some way, steadied her during her ongoing seige of illness—an illness which would flatten most of us once and for all.

A long time ago, years in fact, before I used it as the theme for my first novel, *The Beloved Invader,* I had worked on the truth that God, the Redeemer, *wastes nothing.* Not even one tear.

The idea runs through several of my nonfiction books as well as the novel. It sustains me. I expect it to go on sustaining me.

But when Ruth Vaughn, who has what the world would call "such a tragic illness" tells me, in her lucid way, that she is daily about the business of "proving my belief out"—I am inevitably wonder-struck. In my own lengthening life, I have had many chances to "prove it out" for myself.

Still—nothing has ever wounded me as life has wounded Ruth Vaughn. She causes me to be filled with awe at God's total redemption. She makes me wonder-struck at God Himself.

"Have I understood your philosophy, Genie?" she dared to ask in her letter.

Understood it? She has helped *me* understand it.

Up ahead, in the pages of this book, her readers will *experience*—for her writing is so creative that anyone reading her cannot merely read—he or she must *experience*—the fact of the Redeemer Himself lovingly at work in a shattered human life.

Ruth's extremely rare illness has not caused her to die, but it has caused her to have to learn how to live again in a way so shockingly different, so totally hostile to her dazzling, active, early life that she carries the added burden of grief for the complete loss of every personal dream.

When Ruth Vaughn tells me that, although life has broken apart for her, "I can 'pick up the pieces—put them together again'," I believe her. You will believe her, too, long before you reach the last page of this absorbing, intimate, glowing book.

There are no "pat answers" in it, by the way.

Ruth is not a cliché-flinger.

Ruth is a realist.

What she has found is real. And what you will read are parts of her very private, personal journals where she has recorded the painful realities of "picking up the pieces" of a broken life to "put them together again."

Not to read this book will be all loss.

Having just finished it, I feel as though I should sit down and write a book on what Ruth Vaughn has taught *me*.

—EUGENIA PRICE
St. Simon's Island, Georgia

Preface

"Creative Use"
Has been my Redeemer's goal
Of Unpleasant Circumstance.

"Creative Use"
Has been His yearning
For each tear on my face
    each break in my heart
    each sliver of life-as-I-wanted-it-to-be.

The wisdom gained
The lessons learned
The perceptions found
Overflow in personal journals
Like grain threshed out upon a silo's floor.

Uneven, they are,
As was their painful gathering:
Perceiving, Denying,
Learning, Forgetting,
Exulting, Despairing,
Reaching, Withdrawing,
Rising, Falling,
But
They are my own.
Privately faced.
Personally clutched.
Painfully earned.

13

They are my own
Now hoarded on salt-encrusted pages
Locked in my precious diaries
With my secret key.

Safe.
Secure.
Sterile as stone.

Unbolt the door.
Fling out the windows.
Spread wide the pages.
Let whatever Truth I've found
Open, flow, pour, flood,
Immerse the body and soul
Of whoever reads with needy heart.

Personal learnings are never for one alone:
The seed of the Redeemer God
Must, in every life,
Be resown.

When serious illness jerked me from the brightly colored, joyfully whirling carousel of life-activity and brutally hurtled me into the inky black stillness of an intensive care unit, all my "top-of-the-head, life-through-rose-colored-glasses" theology dissolved like morning mist. I lay desolate.

Isolated in the small cubicle with life-monitoring machines making the only sounds, my sole companions were *questions* . . . screaming, shouting, frantic, ferocious questions . . .

In the first moments, all clichés, all simplistic theories, all pat answers had been marched out and crucified. I could no longer tolerate any concepts that did not square with the stark, painful realities of human life as I now faced them.

Only questions remained.

The questions were no longer theological, theoretical, or sweetly rhetorical. . . . The questions demanded answers with the anguished intensity of a drowning person straining for the life-rope. The questions pounded with panic . . . and I knew that the answers would determine my future and my destiny.

Is there a God?
If so, is He Reliable Reality or Fraudulent Fiction?
If so, WHAT is His Character? Fiend or Friend?
Does God participate in the lives of twentieth-century people?
If so, HOW does He participate?

If so, WHY doesn't His participation deny evil, tragedy, broken-
ness, suffering, life-devastation to His children who try to obey Him?
Does God answer prayer?

If so, does that mean that "Ask and ye shall receive" promises
that my body will be made whole and life-as-I-planned-it will be
returned?
Is God real?

If so, does He care? Even when dreams, plans, hopes are bombed
like Hiroshima and only acrid, mutilated, precious debris remains,
does God care . . . then?

The quest for the answers to these questions began for me in
the black despair of an intensive care cubicle. The quest is one
that all thinking minds must undertake.

This is the record of my quest.

I am indebted to many who companioned me. Three per-
sons especially have had a part in it. The first is a woman whom I
have never personally met. But in my budding maturity, I found
her books. In their pages, I found guidance for building a foundation that held when my life-superstructure was blasted. In her
words, written for the masses, I found a roadmap for personal
understanding.

Her name is Eugenia Price.

Our correspondence began as professionals. To me, as
playwright, she granted the privilege of writing the stage plays of
three of her novels: *The Beloved Invader, New Moon Rising, Light-
house.*

But our relationship deepened into rare friendship. In the
years of this illness, she has been ever *with* me in a multiplicity of
ways: in the creative experiences of transforming her ideas from
novel-narration to drama-action, in steady study of her published
works of exposition, in the private wonder of her letters written
only to me, in gifts, in flowers, even in remarkable poetry such
as:

I love Ruth
In truth!
Forsooth!

She has been my supportive, serendipitous, guiding, guard-
ing, inspiring, inimitable, hand-holding, heart-sharing friend in
The Quest.
But it began long ago.
As a young woman, I systematically, thoroughly studied the
thoughts of Eugenia Price. I can remember walking the floor,
book in hand, straining my brain to understand the concepts she
was stating. Much of it was beyond me then, but the challenge,
the stimulus of her ideas helped me form, even in embryo, my
own philosophy which would emerge slowly in the debris of my
life-dreams.

The second person who impacted this quest was, as you
might suspect, a medical doctor. Dr. Patrick Madden stopped the
clock of his busy professional life to be a personal friend to me
and my family.
He spent hours with each of us, going beyond medical discussions to deal with the raw human agony of life-breaking-apart.
Like Marcus Welby on television . . . he gave full attention to
the total suffering event . . . he displayed compassion for each
personality affected . . . he involved himself personally in The
Quest . . . he stood staunchly with my family and daily gave us
the most beautiful of all gifts: He *cared.*

The third, and most important, person involved in my quest
is my husband, Bill.
We met in a college speech class. I well remember the day. I
stood in the doorway that first class-period and looked over the
group of eligible young men clotted together on one side of the
room. One caught my eye. Thin, blond, dancing blue eyes,
ever-laughing, he reminded me of a long-held dream. My pulse
quickened. Could it be HE?
However . . . playing the role of the coy female, I walked to
sit alone on the *other* side of the room. It was good strategy, I
now know, for he tells me that the conversation had ceased as all

male eyes considered me. But he alone asked: *"Who* is that?"

He was informed of my name and of the current rumor that I was engaged. He had to find out.

So he left his pals and came to sit behind me on the other side of the room. His first words were: "Let me see your left hand."

And when I showed him its diamond-emptiness, he handed me his heart. I accepted with my own return heart-gift.

From that moment, he has been my love.

And when illness shattered the possibility of our pacing together in an active, achieving world, he simply held my hand more tightly and loved me more. On our silver wedding anniversary, our older son, Billy, took one of my book titles to make his point when he said: "You have proven that marriage gets better and better . . . *No Matter the Weather!"*

I did not write this record for publication.

I wrote it as my way of searching for God in the midst of what Emily Dickinson has called "agony absolute." Eugenia Price, Dr. Madden, and Bill all have parts and pieces of this record, written out for them to share my raw human pain.

But the record is an entity in my prolific personal journals. And when I was asked to unlock these diaries for the public, I was uncertain. Edith Hamilton has written: "To suffer is to be alone." And this was my own private battle.

But as I pondered, I understood that although suffering is intensely individual, it is also universal. There are even specific stages in suffering and close, if not identical, healing insights in every person's journey to find God present and sufficient with life-dreams-spurt-apart. To follow these stages in the life of another could be illuminating. To apply healing insights to one's own gaping wounds could speed recovery.

Truth locked up in a personal journal, I perceived, is sterile. It must be opened, spilled, shared so that its treasure of discovery may be valid, vital, viable in transmuting the "agony absolute" of another.

And so I leave my personal record for others who may follow.

And I do so with profound gratitude for three who companioned me . . .

FOR GENIE
My mentor
My guide
My friend
Who challenged my mind
Who comforted my heart
Who charted my path toward the Redeemer God
FOR GENIE
Who cared for me.

FOR PAT MADDEN
My physician
My counselor
My friend
Who went beyond medical jargon
Who filled my cup of quiet
Who pointed to that central stillness
Where wisdom rests.
FOR PAT MADDEN
Who believed in me.

FOR BILL
My husband
My lover
My friend
Who did not run away
When illness left me lying mangled
Midst the broken pieces of my dreams
Who stayed to share
The pain
Of a heart that ached
Of lips that pled
Of eyes that wept
Who solemnly scrutinized
My minuteness
Stripped of
Charm and beauty
Vivacity and sparkle
Talent and achievement
Who touched the secret place
Where I am really *I*
and said
"This is enough.
For you see
It is YOU I love."
FOR BILL
Who loved me.

The Burning Carousel

Life was a carousel!
A glorious whoosh
of a
multicolored
many-splendored
magical-musical
carousel
Who - oo - sh!
The entire atmosphere
of my life
tinkled.
Not softly.
Brightly and clearly
Ringing and joyfully
It tinkled:
Ting, ting, ting,
Ting, ting, - a - ling - a - ling.
The music
Rushed through my life
Like a flitting, flirting breeze
And I would jump on
The whirling horses of adventure
Whee!
Round and round
On the tinseled, shiny hobby-horses of experience
and plop!
I'd jump from one
Landing on my toes
To dance

23

Dance in the joyous excitement of being alive!
Whoosh!
Then with a single bound
I'd leap to another racing ride
Then to another
And another
And another
And - - - - - -
And then
It Stopped!
The Carousel
Stopped!
No more sound of tinkling music.
No more kaleidoscope of bright dizzy colors.
No more giddy laughter.
The World sat on its axis.
The Carousel poised on its platform.
And the sun went out.
The long doors of the dark closed on me.
Although I battered
till my knuckles bled
I was trapped in the midst of storm:
The thunder blared crescendo
As slender streaks of lightning flicked
Like angry whips across the hobby-horse backs
The wind rode by with blatant horn
While great, tall trees of my staunchest faith
Waved like hollow batons
I wept with salty tears of breaking spray
Blown by the roaring fury of the rain upon my face
I yelled, but drowned the sound in pounding storm
I shouted, yet my voice was not my own.
It was the wailing wind and broken pieces of my dreams
Blown in whispering swirls
Around the dead Carousel.

The rain knifed down
My throat was choked and tight
With questions vainly screamed as overhead
The thunder crashed
The lightning struck
And the Carousel was cremated before my stricken eyes
Stripped of all I had known and loved
Bereft of all I had trusted and leaned upon
Denied all my dreams and plans
I stood alone
In the black-enshrouded world
and
cried.

1

Life Isn't Supposed to Be Like This!

It happened to my friend Anna, whose husband divorced her for a younger woman.

It happened to my friend Don, when his only child and heir to his business was killed in an airplane crash.

It happened to my friend Steven, when he was fired from his job with no notice or warning.

It happened to my friend Caryl, when she was held captive for a weekend and raped repeatedly and brutally.

It happened to my friend Jon who, despite his efforts, flunked out of law school.

It happened to my friend Shea, whose facial and physical injuries in an automobile accident ended her career as a model.

It happened to my young friend Burrell, who dove into a lake on a summer day, hit his head on a rock, broke his neck, and will be a quadriplegic for the remainder of his life.

It happened to my friend Cheryl, when she received the news that in spite of their fourteen-room house built for a huge family of children, she was barren.

It happened to my friend Lynn, whose incredible agility on the piano keyboard was stopped by a falling two-by-four that smashed her right hand.

Divorce burned Anna's carousel . . .

Death burned Don's.

Steven was fired; Caryl was raped; John tried and failed.

Shea, Burrell, Cheryl, Lynn stood before their flaming carousels which were set ablaze by physical impairments.

As was my own . . .

The bare facts are that, throughout my life, there were indicators of weakness. Finally, when I was a graduate student at The University of Kansas in 1966, there was such an acute problem that I was hospitalized for diagnosis.

A minor problem was found which could be corrected. But the diagnostician somberly informed me that this only indicated a more serious medical problem looming on my life-horizon, though he was unable to diagnose it at that time.

My body responded to the corrective treatment and I ran back to my carousel, jumped aboard, and roared away with even greater exuberance and joy. I was certain the physician's gloomy forecast was not for the Christian. Whatever had been the problem, I surely was healed, for good health seemed to catapult through my veins.

In 1972, the clutches of the illness began to take firm grip. Through the next two years, a medley of hospitalizations and specialists could do nothing to stay the increasing viciousness of that strangling hold. In 1974, weighing only eighty pounds and with many health problems, I again went to a diagnostic hospital where, on December 1, the elusive diagnosis was made: "Pituitary failure." They told me, "Replacement of the life-essential hormones can give you life, but in limited parameters."

I had not the faintest idea what they meant.

I read their medical textbooks and held long articulate discussions about this strange gland, whose name I had never heard before, and its amazing gifts to the body. The cessation of its function was serious. I could talk knowledgeably about the implications . . . but not one word of it ever applied to *me!*

Because I could discuss the physical limitations so intelligently, my doctor was certain that I understood. So when the body responded to the replacement therapy and stabilized, he said, "You can live a normal life."

He was convinced that I received that word *normal* in light of my perceptive responses to his learned lectures. But he was wrong.

I received the word *normal* to mean the definition of roaring, racing, riotous activity I had always known.

And so . . . from a period of leaking illness, I shot back into life like a team of greyhounds suddenly released at the starting gate. And when I sagged, I lectured myself and rushed on.

For I lived with *contrast.*

When I set life before replacement therapy in juxtaposition with life after, the contrast was a glorious, four-color illustration. I witnessed it with all my senses. Replacement therapy had returned the sparkling glowing *zest* for life! I ignored the fact that the limitations remained.

I look back and marvel at the incredible pace I kept those few weeks back on campus. Replacement therapy had been given to me in rigidly calculated dimensions and I was sternly warned against increasing dosage at any time for any reason.

Extremely conscientious, I did not.

And yet, I changed not a revolution of the speed of my world.

It was totally an exercise of the will. That is all.

I used every erg of energy to roleplay the way I had lived in earlier years. I used every whip of determination to do all the things expected of me.

I claimed no part of the illness. If it came to mind, I shook it away as a "cop-out" thought. I had replacement therapy. *So Ruth, get on with life.*

Deep inside, the clock of mortality began to sound a warning. Tick. Tick. But I did not listen.

As the weeks turned, it began to sound like a gong. TICK. TICK.

I only pushed my life-accelerator harder.

Anything short of giving to my extreme limit every moment of every day was unacceptable to my mind. It had always been. It would always be. The life-essential hormones that could no longer be supplied by my own body were replaced through medication so *all was well.* I focused on that thought and, when the caution bell rang, I plugged my ears, bandaged my eyes, closed the blinds, barred the doors, caulked up the cracks so that its message could not find *any* way to seep in. I was no longer ill.

Life had been returned to me. Life, as I had defined it for a lifetime, was still mine.

So . . . College-teaching, Play-directing, Book-writing, Public-speaking, Student-counseling, Playwriting, Home-keeping, Family-caring, I raced directly into adrenal insufficiency crisis with pituitary insufficiency which medical textbooks say is "fatal in every instance" and I knew, deep inside, that "limited parameters" had not been merely words to use in medical discussions of a fascinating, alien illness. Somehow their tentacles had fastened on *me!*

And the nurses told me that I whispered over and over in my pain: "I can't ever live like that again!"

As my carousel burned around me, I found the Redeemer God *with* me. And the words He spoke, deep inside where the meanings are, were these: "Be of good cheer!"

I screamed at Him: *No! No! I can't! Not this time!*

As a child, I had memorized the words of Jesus recorded in Matthew 14:27. They resounded over the blaze of flaming carousel: "Be of good cheer; it is I, be not afraid."

My shrill laughter at such absurdity shouted back:

But I am afraid! No! I am terrified!

I never knew darkness could be so black!

I never knew fire could be so devastating!

I never knew reality could be so cold!

I never knew destruction could be so total!

I pulled myself taught in my intensity, verbally hurling my agony toward Him: *Don't You know . . . life isn't supposed to be like this!*

Riding on the echo of my sobs were Jesus' words recorded in John 16:33: "These things I have spoken to you, that in me you might have peace. In the world, ye shall have tribulation: but *be of good cheer;* I have overcome the world."

I flung myself earthward in a limp, broken heap: *No! No good cheer! Not now! I never knew a heart could hurt so much!*

I lay inertly like a de-sawdusted doll.

With inner ears, I heard His compassionate Voice:

"Christianity is not a guarantee against such knowledge, Ruth.

"Christianity is a guarantee that I will be with you when you face that knowledge . . . and I will bend with you in *redeeming* the situation . . . if you will allow."

I closed my eyes in wry understanding.

Eugenia Price had taught me well.

Even now, He could speak to me as the Redeemer God . . . Redeemer of sin . . . Redeemer of burned carousels. I understood the theory . . . but it was hopeless.

I looked about at my dark, dank, destroyed world and shuddered.

Redeemer God, I said aloud, *it sounds nice . . . But there is nothing left to redeem.* My eyes took in the scene and understood that life-as-I-planned-it was gone forever, like the ripple on the pond as the pebble sinks, like the mist in the morning. The magical-musical carousel was gone. And the silence was furry and moist and full of claws. I began to weep achingly as I whispered: "There is nothing left."

But His love enwrapped me like flannel as His Inner Voice rang through my spirit:

There is no life so lost that it is irretrievable. .
There is no situation so broken that it is irreparable.
There is no heart so shattered that it is irredeemable.
Trust Me.

Katherine Mansfield wrote: "The little boat enters the dark fearful gulf and our only cry is to escape—'Put me on land again.' But it's useless . . . The shadowy figure rows on. One ought to sit still and uncover one's eyes."

And when one "uncovers one's eyes," and can study the testimony of another who has also journeyed in "the little boat" through "the dark fearful gulf" to find God present and sufficient, it could be invaluable.

With my life-carousel in dead ashes, He climbed into "the little boat" *with* me. He journeyed "the dark fearful gulf" *with* me and, ultimately, He guided my craft to a shore where He enabled me *to create a new world . . .*

A new carousel . . .

Its colors are muted
Its splendors are softer
Its music flows *pianissimo*.

But it is a beautiful carousel with
its own movement
its own tunes
its own adventures.

And I love it.
I wrote in an early journal:

"I shall build for the second half of my life much as I built for the first: creatively, with my whole heart."

I have done that.
This is my personal record, bearing witness for others who may follow.

2

In the
Secret Place

My doctor was kind.

"Life, as you define it," he said, "is impossible."

We looked at each other solemnly.

He had come to know me well.

He had been so impressed with my quick grasp of information, my free-wheeling articulate expression at the time of diagnosis that he had felt secure in my understanding. He thought I felt comfortable with the changes that would have to come in my life.

He had been wrong, and now I could feel the intensity of his concern reaching to me through the silence.

He had listened to my schedule before and admired my abilities. Now he understood their dangers.

He had known what a circus act I made of life. I never walked. I ran, wheeled, spun, whirled through each day, draining my creative springs with little time for refilling. With my pitcher of multitalents, I attempted to daily water a field, not a garden. I threw myself indiscriminately into the rushing, whooshing, dizzying dazzle I called *life!* He had known and rejoiced in my skills and competencies. But he thought we had a clear understanding that I could never live like that again.

Now he knew how wrong had been his assumption.

He looked at me and shook his head. "I can't imagine how

you lived eight weeks," he said. "Your efforts to live like that, in spite of your comprehensive knowledge, leave me bewildered." His voice was gentle with his caring. "Life, as you define it, is impossible."

Was redefining possible?

I could see the doubt in his eyes. I could feel it in my heart.

"Never teach again," he warned. "Never direct another play. Move from the locale where your hyperactive habit patterns are ingrained. . . . And even then . . ."

As he paused, I whispered, "I'll try."

His eyes were warm with his understanding of my earnest promise. "I know you will," he sighed wistfully. "You will try very hard. But even so, you will probably fail, and . . . you will probably die. All your definitions are in the jumping-up-and-down, irrepressibly-in-love-with-life, proceed-with-iron-will-power dimensions."

He leaned back in his chair and studied me carefully. "To redefine the essence of life itself is difficult, Ruth, probably impossible. But it *is* your only chance to live."

When he had gone, I tried to think it through.

The team of doctors had spent hours with me explaining the illness to me at the time of diagnosis. But I had disbelieved that their discussion had anything to do with *my* life.

Perhaps that is common error when the physical problem cannot be *seen*. Had my leg been amputated, I would have believed. But with *unseen* life-essential hormones available in limited amounts of replacement therapy, it was easy to enter their exciting medical discussions, all the time pushing away any thought that inner-amputation was mine.

And the replacement therapy had been exactly as if I had been dead and now, reborn, I could scarcely believe my marvelous good fortune in being alive. I was astonished at the beauty of the world. I was overwhelmed at the remarkable qualities of every person. I was euphoric with resurrection joy.

WOW! Life, I cannot hold you close enough!

Did I really believe *any* of it?

I truly think I did not.

When I was sixteen, I was enchanted with the beauty of Psalm 91. I memorized it and repeated it every night at bedtime.

"He that dwelleth in the secret place of the most High shall abide under the shadow of the Almighty."

In that lovely sentence, I thought I had found a guarantee against all problems of life. I believed it promised all good things from a good tennis backhand to immunity to disaster.

Every psychologist will tell you that one of the basic needs of the human psyche is security. At age sixteen I felt that, in this one psalm, I had a written guarantee for enveloping safety.

My "logic" came from years of Sunday school, thundered sermons, and my own personal experiences with God.

God had been real to me since my earliest memories. As a tiny child, I sang songs with His breezes. I raced through meadows shouting for Him to observe my agility. I read Him my poetry in the top of my beloved mulberry tree. And He listened to me wherever I was.

I told Him about my excitements, my disappointments, my concerns. Although I was the only child at home after my eighth year, I never felt lonely because my Best Friend was always with me.

I knew God personally.

I loved Him dearly.

With every corpuscle of my being, I strove to please Him.

Oh, yes, surely I dwelt "in the secret place of the most High" and I snuggled in the fact that "under the shadow of the Almighty," I was forever secure.

I thought Psalm 91:1 was an equation for triumph:

> God-obedience = plans-fulfillment
> God-love = goals-attainment
> God-partnership = dreams-come-true.

I was wrong.

No such equation is stated or implied. But because I did not understand that, I now confronted the stark suffering of a false belief.

"He that dwelleth in the secret place of the most High shall abide under the shadow of the Almighty."

For a long time, my sixteen-year-old interpretation seemed correct.

It was easy to see God's hand at work shaping my life as the potter shapes the clay on His wheel of destiny.

I married a blond, bouyant, bewitching young man who made all my star-wishes of love come true. I went with him to live in a parsonage where I found fantastic adventure.

I gave birth to two sons who were beautiful, beguiling, beloved.

I hadn't known happiness came in such overflowing measures. Everything was covered with golden splendor.

My professional writing career began at age twenty-one with my first published magazine article. It expanded at age twenty-two with my first published book which kept pace with more than one-a-year. My dream of heart-sharing through words was reality.

A college campus gleamed on our horizon. My husband became chairman of the department of speech communication and I hurled myself into the dazzle of teaching creative writing, drama; directing plays; racing through the world on wings of pure joy.

How easy it was to see God's hand in all that glorious sunshine. Ah! Surely I dwelt in the "secret place of the most High!" Surely I was secure from all alarms "under the shadow of the Almighty!"

I exulted under clear, azure skies.

And then . . . the azure skies blackened, the exultation gave way to pain, and the sun went out . . . But only for a while—only for a while.

For then came diagnosis, replacement therapy, and the incredulity of literal physical resurrection.

In my journal, I wrote:

"A twelve-hour IV," he said.
Strange! I thought. I wonder why.
But I lay back in my dull lethargic nausea, content to let them try any whim that pleased them so long as I did not have to move.
The hours passed uneventfully and the IV was removed. A few

hours went by. Suddenly my eyes opened and I thought: "I'm hungry!"

The thought screeched on hinges rusty from long lack of use.

Surprised, I sat up and examined my sensations. Why, certainly, my stomach was not turning as was usual these days, weeks, months, at the thought of food. In fact, I actually was hungry! I looked about in wonder and was aware of a sudden and incredible sense of well-being, as of new blood, new zest, new joy pouring all through my body. I felt vigorous, excited, challenged with the glory of life. I had not felt like this in months, no, not for years. I looked at the bright light of the evening sun and I knew it had never seemed so sharp, or at least not for a long time. The flowers in the room flooded every inch with fragrance. Had they been this way before and I had not known it until this moment? All of life, suddenly, became quicker, closer, keener, and so very dear, and so filled with peace.

It had been so long since I had felt anticipation and eagerness, yet they were rising in me now, an exultant tide. My fingers shook as I touched my blazing cheeks and whispered, "Thank You, God."

And the tears spilled in a surge of thanksgiving and adoration and humility and joy at the unexplained, incredible storm of life that raced through my veins.

Later, when they explained the problem of cessation of the pituitary gland's function, they said: "Such cessation is always fatal unless replacement therapy is instituted." And now . . . my failing strength was truly being resurrected.

"There are no words sufficient," my heart whispered. I was slowly dying and now I'm given, in one fell swoop, the gift of life. The bright, joyful, bubbling part of me had already died long ago. Now to my total astonishment, she is reborn.

A detached part of me observed that "newly resurrected" person who bounced down hospital hallways, meeting people, laughing, chatting, her eyes sparkling . . . and I remembered (from the far, distant, dusty past) a person like that!

She had died.

Slowly, I had watched her die until I had truly forgotten her. And now as I watched her bounce back in the rebirth of life, I knew my heart was right: there were no words sufficient. I could only look on in total awed wonder and amazement. She, who was dead, was alive!

The body that was dying throbbed with the shock of life reborn.

There were no words sufficient . . . only an incoherent mingling of worship, awe, incredulity, gratitude, joy, and total thanksgiving for the exulting, throbbing gift of life: a miracle.

In my Christmas letter to family and friends that year, I wrote:

"Now that I am home from the hospital, I want to share with you whom I love the news of our joy. I will return to the hospital in six weeks for a check. The body has been severely damaged; I am incredibly weak, but the zest for life is back! How beautiful it is! How I revel in colors I had ceased seeing, music I had ceased hearing, exuberance that had died.

"The entire episode has been a beautiful spiritual experience. I have learned lessons in stillness that would have been impossible with racing feet. And now that life has been given back to me, my happiness is boundless. Every aspect of the universe hits me with reverberating shocks of wonder. I feel in harmony with life, melted into the universe, lost in it, as one is lost in a canticle of praise, swelling from an unknown crowd in a cathedral. 'Praise ye the Lord, all ye fishes of the sea . . . all ye birds of the air . . . all ye children of men . . . Praise ye the Lord!'"

All the medical discussions, all the study of medical textbooks, all the analysis of funny diagrams of the pituitary gland and its functions had been only fascinating new material for discussion. I had met every word of it with *total disbelief* that it had *anything whatever* to do with me.

After the first days back in my dizzying schedule, an inner warning began to sound. I remember dashing out of the dean's office one day, my arms loaded with books, his wife stopped me. "How *are* you?" she asked. I thought I detected a flicker of real concern in her eyes and I laughed. Nervously. For, deep inside, I was unsure.

I was amazed when I confessed: "The exuberance, the excitement, the enthusiasm is *all* back . . . but sometimes my body doesn't know!"

As I rushed on to play rehearsal, I puzzled over my response.

Always positive in my words and thoughts, why had I blurted out this negative? I knew, in a secret compartment rarely consulted, that weakness was beginning to claw again . . . and each day it became more frenzied, more pitiless. But I had not intended to admit the knowledge to myself . . . certainly not to another.

After rehearsal, I drove out to the lake and sat on the grass. A pair of mallards swam slowly by, their feet pushing backward, leaving ripples on the placid water. I had watched them dozens of times in my life . . . dating back to afternoons Bill and I sat on this same spot when we were students in this college. The mallards swam the same; the water moved the same; the air tingled with sweetness the same.

The world steadied and the warning bell hushed. Yellow marsh grass, calm high tide, pale September sky. They were there as they had always been. And the tide would come in tomorrow. The mallards would swim calmly. God was still with me as He had always been.

I could feel Him sitting with me in love. His Presence was such a happy habit I rarely stopped to think about it. He had always been natural with me. I had always been natural with Him. No formality, no Sabbath manner, no strain. Just friends together. And He had said: "Be of good cheer;" "It is I;" "Be not afraid."

Surely I dwelt "in the secret place of the Most High" and was thus secure within "the shadow of the Almighty." I stretched out on the grass in relief. All would still be well.

But it wasn't.

Eight weeks after whirling back onto a college campus, my body went into crisis. And nurses say I whispered over and over what I had suspected in my spontaneous response to the dean's wife: "I can't ever live like that again!"

Now, after surviving that dangerous crisis, my doctor posited the challenge: Redefine the total essence of life . . . or die.

Once, when I was twelve years old, I had stood with my father in a thunderous storm where lightning jumped about like parachutists dropping from the skies. I remember the jarring moment when the small cabin in front of us was struck.

Now, years later, I lay in a hospital bed feeling that same sensation, even the strange acrid smell, the shock of instant destruction. A tremendous flash split my world. The bolt entered the top of my skull as I got the message. I, Ruth Vaughn, had been struck. This illness *was* mine.

And I cried.

Life made no sense.

I could not see God's hand at work.

The azure sky had turned to midnight black.

There was no "secret place of the most High" protecting me from the irrevocable facts of my personal tragedy. There was no "shadow of the Almighty" denying the breaking up of my beloved world.

And I cried.

I was helpless, trapped in the grip of circumstances that I was powerless to change. There seemed no way out of my predicament.

Helplessness is a terrifying thing to most of us. We resist it, deny it, and shout that we are immune to it because we dwell "in the secret place of the most High" and live "under the shadow of the Almighty" . . . but when we are face to face with an ultimate in helplessness, such as an incurable illness that changes everything known and planned for, we can see nothing but tragic waste.

I lived through the following days and weeks in the hospital like a blind person digging in darkness, desperate and alone. Digging for a treasure that had to be there, a treasure I could not find.

But WAIT! WAIT! WAIT!

I had only made a lapse in my faith. I *did* have the treasure!

Oh, yes, surely that was it.

I would simply march up to the holocaust and pour the words of Psalm 91 on the guzzling, gaudy fires of my life-plans . . . and they would be drowned! Isn't that what faith in God meant? Isn't that the treasure?

Of course! Of course!

Laughing in relieved wonder, I stood close to the leaping flames and shouted: "He that dwelleth in the secret place of the most High, shall abide under the shadow of the Almighty."

There!

Wouldn't the onpouring of those words drench the fire?

No.

Instead, the words seemed to crumble into dust as they touched the fire, the orange-tipped flames leaping higher and dancing more exotically.

WHY? WHY? WHY?

My heart screamed with the agony.

Were those words I had repeated every night of my sixteenth year proven to be merely pretty poetry in a promissory note not payable on demand?

Were they only a pious platitude?

Was the Most High only an imagined God, as helpless as a paper tiger?

Was the "secret place" an illusion?

Was the "shadow of the Almighty" a lie?

I buried my face in my hands.

My thoughts fluttered like moths in candlelight. I strained for answers but none came. After a long moment, I pounded my bed with my fists. "I won't settle for theories! I need Truth . . . and I don't know how to find it!"

And so I boarded "the tiny boat" and entered "the dark fearful gulf." And I thought . . . I truly believed in that moment . . . that I was alone.

3

Not Alone

*H*eartbreak.

I'd always thought it a tarnished word from the tabloids or old-time movie magazines I had pored over as a teen-ager: "The real story behind Elizabeth Taylor's . . . Debbie Reynolds' . . . Eddie Fisher's . . . heartbreak!"

But as Bill brought me home following crisis and settled me in my bed, I felt the break literally. The crack was so real it seemed to be something I could see.

Bill had gone to the college and I lay looking out my bedroom window. A strange afternoon it was: the sky was bright yet it was snowing big, fluffy, lazy flakes. I watched them falling softly by my window. My eyes closed now and then. When I opened them, it was with enormous effort. Even breathing tired me. My fingers lay still on the covers.

Suddenly I was back in the top of the mulberry tree where I had spent so many hours as a little girl. It was an amazement. How could I ever have been a little girl in pink ruffled pinafore, careful-mother-finger-shaped curls, singing songs or writing poetry in the open arms of the large brown tree?

But it was true. I could remember the roughness of the bark, the shape of the emerald leaves, the Presence of God with me. I caught my breath.

If God were with me in the mulberry tree, would He not be

with me now? I in-took my breath sharply. My faith was torn up the way a plow tears up a cotton field. Nothing would ever be simple again.

Perhaps never simple again . . . but what about God's Presence?

Does He still companion my life?

"Man is essentially alone," I remembered from some poem.

Was that true? Had the God in the mulberry tree only been a figment of a childish imagination of the same mosaic logic of my black-and-gold Edmund Dulac fairy-tale book where the handsome prince or the beautiful princess always overcame every obstacle to live happily ever after?

Following my thrust into crisis, I remembered, the decision was made to fly me via ambulance plane back to the hospital where the diagnosis had been made. A registered nurse would accompany me, and Bill would come later by car.

When the plane landed, an ambulance screamed me to the emergency room where endocrine specialists waited. But it was a different team. Not one of them had ever seen *me* before. They knew my medical history; they were prepared to try to save my life. But not one of them *knew* me.

Loneliness almost strangled me.

I reached out my hand as my heart whispered with urgent intensity: "Mother!" I knew she was dead.

"Bill!" I knew he was in a speeding car.

"Dr. Thompson!" He, my physician in diagnosis, was not on duty at this time.

My body was struggling between life and death. *And I was alone.*

As I looked at my outstretched pleading hand, an unexplainable warmth brushed it. It was exquisitely gentle and fragile, like the movement of a wind-flower.

In tears of recognition, I knew I was not alone.

Mother was dead. Bill was coming from another state. Dr. Thompson went about other duties.

But God was with me. As He had been with me in the mulberry tree, on a college campus, in riotous activity, He was with me in that emergency room. I knew. I felt. And slowly, very deliberately, I watched as I closed my outstretched hand and pulled it back onto the stretcher.

As I slipped again into unconsciousness, I was securely aware that I *was* companioned. I was not alone.

Now back in my home, as I looked out at the bright blue square of sky dropping snow, I believed God sat with me then. "Blessed are they that mourn: for they shall be comforted."

I was in mourning. How I could find comfort, I had not one clue. But at least I was not deserted.

Claiming the peace of the emergency room, I deliberately folded my hand into a baby-fist and went to sleep. Pain waited for me when this hour was over. I understood that. I would have to find an answer to the problem of human suffering. My "little boat" was adrift on the "dark, fearful gulf" where I would have to confront the truth of the relation of God to human need.

But for now, I would simply trust Him.

Like the little girl of long ago, I would relax in my *assumption* of God's love for me. For now I would just believe that He held my hand.

The next days ran together. There was no morning, no afternoon, no day or night. There was only sleep. Beautiful, delicious, healing sleep.

Gradually, strength began to return. And small blocks of time when I lay awake, pondering the beauty of the world outside. There were times of blazing, brilliant sunshine in a cobalt sky. Even nearing December, some of the trees were still on fire. Now and then a few leaves drifted by my window like yellow sparks to lie on the dark pebbles of the rock garden.

I know I may be dead soon, I thought. *But that's not the point. What counts is right now. I've got this moment, this cupful of beauty.* Tears would surface from awe and wonder as my love for the world overflowed and splashed all around the room.

I turned, in habit, to thank God . . . and that gave me a view of the waiting questions. But I had not the strength to face them.

I knew I would not find the answer in submission. That was Islam.

I knew I would not find it in merely resolving to go on with life as I understood it. That was Stoicism.

I had long ago decided that truth did not lie in those poles of thought. But where then? If God is love and omnipotence, then is He responsible for burned life-carousels, the destruction of dreams, the shattering of human hearts? And if He is responsible, then He is a Fiend and there is no sanity in trusting Him and no comfort in His Presence.

I had no strength to reach for the answers.

I could not bear to ask Him to leave me.

And so my heart would whisper: *O why don't You right my world with a physical healing? Why don't You give me a quick happy miracle: "And she lived happily ever after?"*

My eyes filled with tears as my heart bulged with pleading: *O why don't You explain Yourself to me? In the mulberry tree, it was all so simple. And now I cannot understand. I cannot. I hurt myself with these thoughts because I am not strong enough to think clearly. So I must leave them. I must let them go for now.*

But God . . . don't leave me. Whatever I find of You in later study . . . for now, God of the mulberry tree, wait with me. Wait, wait with me.

And He did.

The calendar pages flipped into the Christmas season. At a youth party, my fourteen-year-old Ronnie's youth leader asked his group a thought-provoking question. He said: "I want you to think carefully over this year. Select the one most important thing that happened to you, the one thing that will affect your life the most."

When Ronnie told me of the incident, I wondered if he had named being elected to the student council, winning the golf tournament, or getting his football letter. But he by-passed all these splendid things and said: "God let my mother live."

I was swaddled in his love.

On Christmas Day, we opened our gifts. When it was all over, twenty-year-old Billy came to us. He shifted his feet awkwardly and said: "I don't know how to say this in writing . . . or how to wrap it up like something for the tree . . . so I'll just do it right out: This is for you."

He shoved a piece of paper into my hand and when I opened it, it was a check made out to Bill and Ruth Vaughn for one hundred dollars. I looked at my collegiate son in astonishment and he said hurriedly: "Don't say a word! I know how expensive hospitals are. I just want to do my part."

I turned to Bill with brimming eyes. Tears splattered his cheeks as he said: "He has the right. He earned the money. It's his . . . and he loves you too."

I was blanketed in his love.

The three men knelt then by the sofa on which I lay. Each boy held a hand; Bill cradled my head in his palms as he said to God: *As we have approached this moment, we have been acutely aware of how different Christmas would be for us if You had not given us the miracle of Ruth's return to life . . .*

And we all wept in gratitude . . .

Gratitude for all that we had almost lost, for all that we had never really seen before . . .

Gratitude for the little things, like the aroma of turkey in the oven, the warmth of the carpet to bare feet . . .

Gratitude for the special things, like the tall bedecked tree, the sound of carols softly sung on the stereo . . .

Gratitude for all the big things, like birth and love and death; for this world and other worlds; for the flesh and for the spirit; for the moment and for eternity; for the miracle of prayer and the presence of God.

In the flood of our shared tears, Bill kissed me and I was enveloped in his love.

We clung together that Christmas morning, the four of us, in such worshipful thanksgiving that I could only raise my thin, quavery voice in the words of the old hymn:

> What a Friend we have in Jesus
> All our sins and griefs to bear
> What a privilege to carry
> Everything to God in prayer.

Our voices joined together in affirmation of our belief in the abiding Friendship of Jesus. We all knew that my "little boat" . . . and theirs all tied with mine . . . were journeying in a "dark, fearful gulf" where we had never been before. We had no desire to be there now. But "the shadowy figure" rowed on.

We did not know the future. But in that moment, we knew the Divine Presence was with us.

4

God!
Explain Yourself!

Christmas transformed into a new year.

Strength began to return to me and I gradually understood that the time had come, as Katherine Mansfield wrote: "to sit still and uncover one's eyes." I had evaded the closets of questions long enough.

Over and over, in my personal journals of that period, I wrote: *Don't fight a fact, Ruth. Deal with it.*

Fact: Life, as I defined it, was over. My carousel had burned.

Fact: Bill would resign from the college to move me to a place where my hyperactive habit-patterns were not ingrained. His career in this place was over.

Fact: My children's home in this locale was uprooted forever.

Fact: Even though my physician recommended the move, they predicted that I would die soon anyway . . .

Fact: I prayed for a miracle.

Fact: *Nothing happened.* Nothing . . . at all.

Don't fight a fact, Ruth. Deal with it.

I paced the floor in my throbbing torment.

I scolded God like a shrew.

I demanded explanation, justification, miracle . . . and all I met was a vast silence.

Why? Why? Why? I demanded. *Is it because You have no explanation, no justification, no miracle? God! Explain Yourself!* . . . *if You can!*

And when there was no divine answer, no thunderbolt of justification . . . when there was no miracle, a spasm of suffering grabbed me and shook me like a dog shakes a rabbit.

I honestly tried for rational, even detached, thought . . . pushing the pain of loss back in my mind until it would recoil and jump back at me . . . not true, clear, calm . . . but the pendulum would swing too far and I would be caught in uncontrollable gusts of grief that left me depleted.

Don't fight a fact, Ruth. Deal with it.

My *fact* was that my life-carousel was burned.

And there was not *one* word from God as to *why!*

I wrote in my journal:

Here I stand in the midst of destruction. Dreams toppled, goals reduced to rubble, the struts and props of life-as-I-planned-it heaving, groaning, collapsing. The blitz is impulsive, wanton, random, and ruthless. To look at it with clear eyes does not imply an acceptance of its desirability. It is starkly admitting that I belong to what has been destroyed, and to pretend otherwise is both foolish and contemptible.

My God, I've "uncovered" my eyes; I'm looking at reality. WHY won't You explain it to me? WHY won't You justify such waste? WHY won't You work a miracle to make the world-all-right again?

It was aphotic night for the soul. I was lost in the darkness of change. And God was silent.

I have loved You. I have believed in You. I have lived for You. I have been willing, if necessary, to die for You. Beyond this, the responsibility is Yours. You created the world and all in it. And You created me so that I lack the capacity to SEE in the dark. God! Explain Yourself!

And I huddled, a mangled, mottled mess on the floor, "lost in the darkness of change" . . . lost in a vast silence.

I was sucked ferociously into this whirlpool of doubt on the dark journey. It would be a long time before my "little boat" would be able to get free.

Another vicious trap which threatened to capsize my "little boat" was the dire fear that God was silent because He did not care.

This is where I hurt the worst.

Although my mind longed for explanations, my whole being yearned chiefly to know that God *cared!* In spite of howling cynicism, I still understood, deep inside, that Christianity is a *way of living* that relates time to eternity, history to truth, a way by which God appeared in the flesh of a Man and a Man was crucified because He was God. I knew that my faith was less something to be understood . . . as one understands why three plus three makes six . . . than something to be *experienced* . . . and then verified through the actual process of living. . . . But that was all dependent upon a God who cared enough to offer Himself in sacrifice for His own creation . . . who deeply, totally, completely, incredibly, *cared.*

My mind wanted answers to questions. That whirlpool still rocked my "little boat" . . . but the most fearful ravage came in the suction: *Are You silent because You simply do not care?*

I might not have fallen so deeply into this trap had it not been for the terrible shock of the speed with which telegrams, flowers, and letters of condolence came in. I was astonished that everyone so calmly accepted the fact of my life-breaking-up.

So quickly, so easily, without a murmur of protest, without one rebellious "It cannot be!", the people in my exterior world seemed to believe that life as I had planned it was gone from me forever . . . and so what else is *new?*

Like front-page news, I was to discover, wreckage must be new to be interesting. A six-month-old heap of debris once a glowing life-carousel (blasted by divorce, death, bankruptcy, illness, whatever) is scarcely worth a second card or flower. Oddly enough, the tragedy of a personal blitz is rarely real for onlookers.

That sounds so harsh that I, on the outside of others' sorrows, want to mute it, change it somehow. But I think it is fact. Once the "little boat" enters the "dark fearful gulf," there is an essential human loneliness, for it *is* an individual journey. Others are wending their own, often torturous ways and so we make our way alone with God . . . for there *is* an unrelenting reality that other human beings do *not* companion us in "the little boat."

As is true in most, if not all, cases of life-spurting-apart, so it was in mine. There was the flurry of acknowledgment of my destroyed world, the courtesy of sympathy extended, and unflurried acceptance.

I was staggered. The mere thought of such a fact in my world was not only unacceptable; the serene admission of it seemed heretical.

I think it was extreme in my case. I had always been strong, resilient, smiling. Those onlooking assumed I would continue to be strong, resilient, smiling. And so they calmly moved on with their lives.

That it *is* that way for others is borne out in the mail that floods my house detailing holocaust. That it *was* that way for me is borne out in a note written to me by my brother only last week, years after the initial blow. He penned: "As I share some of your life-experiences with others, I face again how glibly we force ourselves to accept life-leveling circumstances in the lives of others, because it hurts us too much to be directly involved."

I think that a fair appraisal of what happens.

No matter the cause of "life-leveling circumstances in the lives of others," people will engulf the wounded one in only the first days when they falsely assume that grief is the worst. That, of course, is not true because one is, at first, blessedly anesthetized with disbelief.

What is true is that it is not for the moment one is struck that one needs hand-holding caring, but for the long journey through "the dark fearful gulf." The long journey that truly seems to have no end.

As I have pondered this reality, I have concluded that it is human nature to get off the duty gesture of sympathy as quickly as possible because that action releases the sender from having to be involved longer in the suffering of the wounded person. We feel helpless, uncomfortable, even afraid when confronted with destruction of another's world, whatever its cause, because that confrontation makes us acutely aware of our own susceptibility. We want to get away from such thoughts, so we do our duty with a flower or card and try to forget the pain of another.

People wrote to tell me: *"I* know you're adjusting wonderfully" . . . "You're such an inspiration to *me"* . . . "Thank you for going through all of this with such strength and beauty so *I* can learn from you" . . . *"I* feel so badly this has happened to you" . . . *"I* know this is going to be a wonderful spiritual experience" . . .

The general essence of people's responses to me was a focus on themselves . . . and the certainty that I was sitting in the midst of life-debris smiling until my lips cracked!

I wondered why then. I may know the answer now.

I believe that self-focus alleviates our need to truly *look* at the pain the other must be feeling. I believe that the triumphant clichés help us deny our own vulnerability to world-blasting. The kind of response I received was (unconsciously) designed to keep my friends from dealing with the realities of their own fragility. Life-worlds so easily explode through illness, death, divorce, and all the other kinds of dynamite that I have come to believe that the fear of really facing that reality for self outweighs the desire of most of us to help another.

I wish my friends had written with loving comprehension of the fact that I was in raw agony, deep distress, a whirlwind of turmoil. I wish they could have looked at those wounds and addressed themselves to *me*, a person in pain, rather than *self*-focus on their confidence of my joy in the midst of this "great spiritual experience."

I wish they had *not* written in clichés about how spring follows winter. I was *in* winter and it did not comfort me in the slightest to know that spring would follow. I was living in the present that consumed my every heartbeat with throbbing torment and I had *no* interest in pious platitudes about what was to come . . . some day! When one is in great pain, one cares only for the moment and how to possibly survive it. Clichés are like rusty hooks in the spirit.

I wish someone had dealt with the *truth*. I wish someone

had said: "Now, Ruth, what has happened to you is a very bad thing." I wish they had not gloried in my pain as something wonderful because it could teach them or me wonderful insights. I lived in the reality of a tragedy. I needed someone to honestly share that reality with me.

I wish someone had written me that it is proven fact that grief over the loss of a beloved world moves in stages and there must be time for mourning. I now know that studies prove there is a pattern to grief. I did not know that then. I believe that had someone cared to share that with me, it would have been helpful. It would not have lessened my present pain, but it would have given me hope.

Elizabeth Kubler-Ross has done excellent research on death and she says there are five steps for a person's accepting his imminent death. I found them similar, if not identical, to the ones I, and others, go through in accepting life on the other side of broken dreams. They are: denial, anger, bargaining, depression, acceptance. I wish someone had told me that.

I wish someone had asked me *how it felt to be me in those circumstances*. Not one person did. Not one person wrote me the question: "How do you feel?"

It would have been my greatest release to pour out my heart to someone who really cared. I could do that to my family, to my physician. But there is something imperative about finding a friend *outside* the family who wants to know and share the pain.

Courage and gallantry. That is what people wanted to believe of me. It is a rare soul who will walk past that façade to reach in *to* the frightened weeping person inside . . . whose life has just split apart.

I reached out. One time. To my best friend.

She had known me as the strong, smiling, creative spirit whose laughter sparkled sunshine all over her life. When I telephoned her, I burst into tears when she answered. Immediately I could sense her embarrassment. Her uncertainty. Her unease.

She had no idea what to say.

And as I understood, I pulled myself together and we ended the conversation with a lot of funny memory-anecdotes and much nervous laughter.

I hung up the phone and sat long, head on the desk, feeling my sense of betrayal. I had, for the first time in our relationship, reached out to her in weakness. She had pulled back in discomfort.

She did not recognize me. She was the one who applauded my strengths; she rejoiced in my achievements; she laughed with delight at my awards. She simply did not know what to do with me as a hurting human being, flooding tears.

And she was my best, my very best, friend.

And then I had an insight: Each of us goes through life trying to do a creditable job under difficult situations. Each of us has our own capacities for understanding, for expression, for sharing.

My friend had never had the gift of words. She *cared* that I hurt. I believed that. But she was incapable of giving me what I needed in that moment. It was beyond her personal ability.

I could demand it and, when it was not forthcoming, I could end the friendship. Perhaps that could be justified because she met me only in my strength.

Or I could understand.

I could understand that I wanted my friend to respond to me the way my mother would have responded. She could not do that. She was not my mother. She did not know the words.

And so, still sitting with my head on the desk, I made a choice. I chose not to expect from her or ask of her what she could not give. Our friendship remained close until the time of her death, but she never again confronted me in tears. She never again knew I had any moments of sorrow or weakness.

We had built our friendship in another dimension: I, the strong; she, the supportive one who rejoiced in my strength. To turn the friendship around was beyond her capacity. She could *not* be the strong one meeting me in weakness. I understood, forgave, and went on with life.

As I have pondered this torture point, I have since tried to be sensitive to others whose "little boat" enters "the dark, fearful gulf" for whatever reason. Often, I do not reach out at all in the initial flurry of sympathy-giving. I wait until I realize the mailbox is now empty, the floral arrangements have withered and died, and "outside people" have returned to their own lives.

And then I write to say: "I have been in that 'little boat' and I know how dark and fearful is that gulf-journey and I will share it with you *for as long as it takes.*"

Recently, I wrote what my friend, who had just experienced the death of her first child, calls my "redundancy letter." In part, it reads: "I'm just reaching out to hand-hold. I want to tell you that my loving prayers enfold you . . . that I care . . . that I hurt with you. I *am* with you in spirit.

"I am believing in our heartbond enough to believe that you know you need *never* write me if that seems best . . . I understand all kinds of feelings . . . but I do want to also tell you that I am here . . . if and when you need to verbalize over and over and over and over and over and over and . . .

"Please never feel hesitant for fear of being redundant. Pain *is* redundant; ongoing; unceasing; and the cries for help cannot be original or new. The loss is ever the same. The sorrow ever the same. The picking-up-the-pieces is picking up the *same* pieces of the *one* shattered life-dream. So the suffering *is* redundant and I understand all about that.

"Please know you can say whatever, whenever to me . . . and I will understand with *no judgment whatever* . . . just understanding what it's like to be in grief . . .

"I have no pat answers . . . to the problem of grief. It has to be lived through moment by excruciating moment. And my best gift to you is to quietly hand-hold in the pain . . . being *with* you in deep supportive caring, knowing you WILL come through . . . also knowing that certainty does not change *one iota* the degree of your torture now!

"I love you. I care.

"Please use me as a sounding board whenever you have that need. I know about pain. I understand. I hurt with you."

No one wrote me that kind of letter. Just as I never wrote anyone else that kind of letter prior to my own-world-burning-down.

Instead, after the gestures of sympathy whirlwinded about me, outside people (to use my brother's words) "glibly" accepted my life-leveling circumstances because they did not care enough to be "directly involved."

And so . . . I had to ask from my shuddering, sobbing, solitary heap: *God . . . are You now silent . . . because You simply do not care?*

My brother, in his recent card, went on to say: "Ever since I called you the other morning, when I was traveling from New York to Boise, your breaking voice keeps coming to my consciousness, and I realize anew how brave you have been as you live out the tragedy in your life."

Yes. That was my reality.

Other people could come or go. *I*, alone, had to "live out the tragedy" in my personal life.

That was my fact.

And I could not but wonder if God then *cared.*

5

Who Is the Most High?

My mind was heavy, tear-swollen, blank.
Emily Dickinson had understood for she had written:

> Pain has an element of blank;
> It cannot recollect
> When it began, or if there were
> A day when it was not.
> It has no future but itself,
> Its infinite realms contain
> Its past, enlightened to perceive
> New periods of pain.

Slowly, as if words were written on a scroll, my mind unreeled the words: "He that dwelleth in the secret place of the most High shall abide under the shadow of the Almighty."

The melody of the words was cooling and it lay, like a poultice, on my wounded mind. When I had screamed them before my burning life-carousel, it had seemed they were wrapped around a hollow reed, skillfully served up, but unnourishing, like circus cotton candy. Words proceeding from a void into a vacuum.

Now, in this moment of quiet, it seemed that those phrases memorized my sixteenth year might provide the framework, the scaffolding on which to build a new understanding of God.

After a moment, I sat up and asked with clarity: *Who are You, the "most High?"*

I suddenly knew that was the question with which I had to begin. My simpering sarcasm would get me nowhere.

My self-pity was a dead-end street.

I must understand *who* is the "most High"!

And there was a ready answer.

"A Fiend!" my rebellious mind exclaimed. "Any Creator who gives the exuberant zest for life and allows it to be housed inside a fragile body is a Fiend!"

I recoiled. I reached for a pillow and put my head under it.

I knew that wasn't Truth.

I must understand who is the "most High!"

"The Author of Frustration," announced Logic. "That is the only possible conclusion. If, indeed, God guided my life through degree programs to academic expertise . . .

"If, indeed, He guided my life through years of exciting work to give me experiential expertise . . . and then as I reached my prime, He entrapped all of that inside a damaged body so that it is of no use to anyone . . . the only logical answer is that His goal is spiteful frustration!"

It did make sense.

I threw aside the pillow and went to study my reflection in the mirror. I looked at the petite brown-haired figure. *Who* was the "most High" in whom she had always believed?

There was real anguish in her eyes. I could see the pain swell and deepen until finally it seemed as if the eyes and everything around them had vanished and I was looking at nothing but the pain. It was a strange sensation; I felt as if another kind of vision had emerged . . . and I knew that, even in all that pain, the answer of Logic was absurd!

That young woman in the looking glass had a lifetime *relationship* in which to find the answer to this search. And the relationship had not been with a Fiend! Nor with the Author of Frustration. That much I knew experientially and positively.

And so I asked my reflection: "Who is the 'most High?'"

And immediately came the answer.

In a split-second reply, as if waiting in the wings, I heard my own voice repeating words formed in a lifelong relationship. I said: "The 'most High' is a Redeemer God who, if I permit, will enable me to make creative use . . . even of all this!"

Incredulously, I stared at the woman in the mirror.

I was wiser than I thought.

None of my life-shattering made any human sense. I had no idea *how* my faith could be true. But that it *was* my faith, I did not doubt.

I turned and went to the sofa. I picked up my Bible and opened it to the flyleaf where I had articulated the essence of my belief long ago. I looked at the spidery-scrawled words . . . and remembered:

It was a small hospital room.

It had a narrow hard bed, bilious green decor, and outrageously blah pictures. I, the hyperactive graduate student, was still. For one of the few times in my life to that point, I was quiet.

It was fall, 1966, and it was important.

Something was wrong with my body. Now, following days of extensive testing, my physician had promised a report.

The moments dragged, as might heavy seaweed pulled underwater.

Finally I got out of bed and walked to the window.

Outside, people were walking around free under the blue afternoon sky. I could see flashes of bright dresses, the dashing cartwheels of children on the sidewalk. It seemed astonishing that life was going on out there while I stood here, a million miles away, in a hospital room. Waiting.

For what . . . I knew not.

When the door opened, I wasn't ready.

With a sharp intake of breath, I climbed back into bed. Somehow I wished it were still morning.

He did not have a diagnosis. He had some clues. And the somberness of his voice, the gravity in his eyes underlined his prognosis that severe problems loomed on my horizon.

After he left the room, I grabbed my Bible and a pen and wrote on the flyleaf these words:

> When Christ dwells in me, then the ground on which I stand is holy ground because He is standing on it too. And because He is a Redeemer God, He will enable me to make creative use of all, even unpleasant, circumstances.

Now . . . nine years later . . . with the forecast proven, with the elusive diagnosis made, with a body damaged by my own disbelief of reality . . . I reread those words.

I smiled ruefully.

I had no idea, when I wrote those words, *how unpleasant* circumstances could be!

I looked at the spidery-scrawled words. I knew, that, even in my ignorance of burned-carousels, I had been accurate in my faith.

"He that dwelleth in the secret place of the most High shall abide under the shadow of the Almighty."

Who is the "most High"?

He is a Redeemer God who . . . if I choose to *allow* . . . will enable me to make creative use of all, even unpleasant, circumstance. Even serious illness that sets fire to my magical-musical carousel. Because of the years of our *relationship* (from Mother's lullabies through mulberry-tree-songs-and-poetry through fulfilling maturity), I believed that to be true.

I gasped as a batwing of insight dipped inward.

Wisdom is . . . *trusting* the Redeemer God. Wisdom is . . . deliberately looking at self, starkly withdrawn into a tightly-curled ball of screeching suffering, and exercising my power of choice. Wisdom is . . . opening the clenched tentacles and asking the Redeemer God, the "most High," to enable me to make creative use out of what seemed to be total senseless waste!

"Tell me *how* the broken pieces of your life-dreams can possibly be of any use to you now?" leered Logic. "Show me how your expertise in your careers . . . more, show me how your personal life itself will not be total senseless waste. Explain to me."

My brows knit.

"I can't," I answered honestly. "But I *do* believe that God will not waste anything if I give Him a chance to redeem it. I believe He is standing with me in this moment, inviting me to let Him have my grief . . . and trust Him to make something useful, something creative . . . *even now.*"

"And you call that Truth?" sneered Logic.

"I bet my life on it," I asserted with all the thunder I could muster. "It is one thing to believe Truth in abstract terms as I have done all these years. It's something else again to *trust* it."

I took a deep breath.

"Well, here is my chance to trust it, to prove it on out. And I shall. I claim this moment that the Most High is a Redeemer of circumstance as well as of sin. I dare to believe in the midst of the acrid debris of my dreams and plans that God will not waste a single life-sliver if I give Him the chance to redeem."

I can remember the occasion perfectly. I walked to stand in the patio door. The light of the setting sun slashed the wooden fence, so that it was half gilded and half in shadow. Suddenly I realized with a tremendous feeling of exultation that this golden light of the sun, the fragrance of early winter evening, my certainty that God *cared* was a moment of special significance. Whatever was or would be, I participated in this moment of all-embracing beauty and felt a oneness with God.

It was a turning point.

No matter the debris of the past, no matter the dismal prospects of the future, I asserted in that moment that God companioned. More, God *cared*.

There is a mystery, I began to perceive, whose key cannot be fully known to mortal men, only dimly glimpsed by them in rare moments. All we know or ever can know is that in the mystery, God exists . . . And He personally *cares*.

Pascal had said it when, throwing out a lifeline to skeptical minds, he asserted that whoever looks for God has found Him. It is that incredible discovery that is the important one.

"God! Explain Yourself!" I had screamed as my "little boat" wound its way on the "dark, fearful gulf."

He had not.

But I now knew *who* He was.

And so I was willing to trust Him to show me How He could make creative use of . . . even a burned, beautiful, beloved life-carousel.

In the "little boat" on the "dark, fearful gulf," I would take abstract Truth and prove *if* it were worthy of my trust. I bet my life that it would be.

I wrote in my journal:

I have chosen my Guide. I will follow Him, hoping to have sufficient courage not to lose heart, sufficient sense not to allow myself to be confused or deflected from my purpose, and sufficient faith to follow Bunyan's advice and endure the hazards and humiliations of the way because of the worth of the destination.

The "most High" was in "the little boat" with me.
I could wait.

6

The Stiff
Heart Questions

*F*aith, I think, is seldom cut and dried. It ebbs and flows, advances and recedes, rises and falls. One's spirit may reach serenity in one moment and plummet into numbness in another.

I wrote in my journal:

I am in a kind of stupor now. I do not go into my office or think of the college. I don't even like to hear Bill talk about his activities there. I escape such conversations whenever I can.

That world is gone for me. I'll never teach another class. I'll never direct another play. I'll never counsel another student. I can't get it back by thinking of it. It is gone—that world. There is nothing to do. How futile to try to hang on to it by scraps.

Bill has resigned. He will move me to another world where doctors say I will die. They tell me to redefine life, and I have not the vaguest notion what they mean. They tell me to live within "narrow parameters." The only image that gives me is of the small pen one makes in which to place a goose for fattening for Thanksgiving Day. I rather understand that image. I do feel much like a goose!

Don't fight a fact, Ruth. Deal with it.

And I do. I prepared myself academically, experientially to be a college professor and dramatist for a lifetime. Just as that carousel was tinkling most delightfully, I was jerked off it and told to 'live like a goose' or die.

*That sounds bitter. I'm sorry. I don't think it is bitterness really.
I feel absolutely numb.*

Emily Dickinson understood. She wrote:

> After great pain a formal feeling comes—
> The nerves sit ceremonious like tombs;
> The stiff Heart questions—was it He that bore?
> And yesterday—or centuries before?
> . . . .
> This is the hour of lead
> Remembered if outlived
> As freezing persons recollect
> The snow—
> First chill, then stupor, then
> The letting go.

I believe that this stage on the dark, fearful gulf is partly physical protection. Great sorrow, for whatever reason, is too painful to take in one bitter dose. It would overwhelm. And so we intake bit by bit, in tiny insights, in waves that our minds cannot tolerate for long.

The numbness allows the pain to filter through the soft vulnerable tissues of the spirit slowly so that it does not rip too far too quickly. But there were times when my thought processes pushed past the dispassion, stubbornly like a weed that has been plucked over and over and always bobs back . . . and in those moments, my journal entries dealt with the answers I had to find.

Psalm 91:1 was my structure in much of my search. I had so snuggled in it when I was sixteen that I felt it imperative to study it now. Had I nightly quoted Truth I misunderstood? Or had I memorized a beautifully poetic lie?

Although I often shrank from looking at it, I felt that, to be honest, my quest had to work through this psalm. I had felt so warm, so secure, so serenely confident of this guarantee of my personal pleasure and prosperity that I had to try to understand *why* my simple definition had not worked out in actuality.

I had settled *who* was the "most High." As best I understood I had tried to live a "righteous life" . . . which assured me of dwelling in "the secret place of the most High." Didn't it?

Obviously not.

So when I looked at Psalm 91:1, I felt stunned astonishment, surging anger, and uncomprehending bewilderment.

"He that dwelleth in the secret place of the most High shall abide under the shadow of the Almighty."

Now life had blasted the rosy equation offered me at age sixteen:

Righteousness = Success, felicity, bliss

And as I looked about me, I understood that the reverse equation, that seemed inherent, was not operant either:

Unrighteousness = Failure, adversity, and tribulation

I wrote in my journal:

What, then, is the "secret place of the most High?"

If it were reality, it surely has nothing to do with my previous interpretation. For I have, as honestly as I could, loved and served God with every erg of energy, every moment of time, every beat of my heart . . . surely that would connote righteousness. But as I stand in the ruins of life, as I had planned it, I know that I am not receiving success, felicity, or bliss.

One of my colleagues in my graduate program is an atheist who proudly boasts of his "unrighteousness." He not only lives it; he makes a point of it.

And yet his life is not beset by failure, adversity, or tribulation. Racing in good health, he is achieving dizzying pinnacles we both dreamed of in graduate school. All planned approaches to those pinnacles are now denied me.

So.

Exploded are the pink-tinted equations with which I defined "the secret place of the most High" when I was sixteen. What is the realistic definition? The TRUE definition? I want nothing less. But how, in this impenetrable blackness, can I find it?

The great majority of mankind, I believe, are content with appearances as though they were realities and more influenced by things that seem to be or they want them to be than by things that are. I don't want that. I want only bedrock, unshakable faith.

I believe that faith, like a mountain, is seldom won by frontal assault, however determined or spirited. Instead, one clambers about the circumference, searching out a support here and toehold there. Occasionally the climber pulls himself up to a slightly more elevated plateau where the clouds are less dense and the summit less hidden. But no less often, he slips back, clawing at loose shale in search of a grip, sometimes finding a stay and sometimes plunging into a chasm of doubt from which there seems no way back up.

When I had understood that God *was* with me and *cared* about my pain, I gained a vital toehold that started me up the mountain of faith. But as I scrambled for higher ground, my fingers slipped and I plunged into a cleft so deep that I put my journal aside. For "pain has an element of blank" and I could not think.

I huddled there, in the chasm where I had fallen, and begged for words. *God! Explain Yourself! Where is "the secret place of the most High?"* And the words rode back to me on echoes in the black velvet night.

Emily Dickinson phrased it:

> I shall know why, when time is over,
> And I have ceased to wonder why;
> Christ will explain each separate anguish
> In the fair schoolroom of the sky.
>
> . . . .
>
> I shall forget the drop of anguish
> That scalds me now, that scalds me now.

But the thought of future comfort did not change the "scalding, anguished" present.

And so I crouched in my "separate anguish" like a pricked balloon. Deflated. Defeated. Despairing in the ruins of all my life-understandings . . . with God . . . with God . . . *with* God! Suddenly I jumped to my feet as the impact of the insight hit me full blast. I lifted my face, tears streaming, and whispered in awe:

"The 'secret place of the most High' is . . . *His Presence* . . . in *all* of life: Wherever, however, whenever . . . in *all* of life's changing seasons: *His Presence.*"

I grabbed my Bible and explored those words written in a flash of perception years before:

✝ *When Christ dwells in me, then . . . the ground on which I stand*
is holy ground because He is standing on it too.

"That's it!" I whispered in wonder, in worship.

"That's it! The 'secret place of the most High' *is* . . . the
'holy ground' of *wherever I am!* Holy ground because 'He is
standing on it too' whether it be the dizzying dazzle of a whirling,
splendid carousel . . . or whether it be the hot acrid ashes of a
burned carousel . . . *'holy ground because He is standing on it too!'*

"The 'secret place of the most High' is the 'holy ground' of
wherever I am."

I went out on the patio and crawled up on the table. My
mind was racing . . . reeling . . . leapfrogging back through the
Old Testament record of the God/man relationship. The "most
High" was *with* His children . . . when they were obedient and
loving . . . when they were rebellious and hostile . . . when they
writhed in the agony of suffering wrought by natural law and free
choice . . . God was *with* them.

And, in the New Testament, when Jesus Christ broke into
the pages of history, He entered *into* human life. He, who came
to show men what God is like in its most startling clarity, participated *in* human existence broadly. He hungered; He wept;
He knew friendship; He knew disillusionment; He knew a child's
joy; He experienced a man's anguish, crying, "My God, my God,
why hast Thou forsaken me?" (Matt. 27:46). Jesus Christ lived,
loved, suffered, died . . . participating in the entire human dimension *with* us.

I repeated from memory the scrawled words in my Bible:

When Christ dwells in me, then the ground on which I stand is
holy ground because He is standing on it too.

Inside, I became very still.
Hushed.
I knew I was not headed for Damascus. There was no
blinding light, no all-sufficing phenomenon of tangible divine
Presence, no voice from on high speaking my name.
I perceived my destination was Emmaus and I recognized

the Stranger walking with me. *Walking with me.* In that phrase lay my miracle.

There were no words. No explanations. No justifications.

I had discovered no clues as to why I had to spend the rest of my earthly life inside a damaged body. I had received no promises that the body would miraculously be made whole and life-as-I-wanted-it returned to me. I had experienced no divine revelations, theological explanations, surprising inspirations, or dramatic miracles . . . and yet . . . the inner seething had calmed.

For the first time since a doctor's words set fire to my life dreams, I felt the blanketing warmth of total security. There was no rational reason for it.

I knew the pituitary gland was unchanged.

I knew my carousel of life-plans was in ashes.

I knew, in spite of the move from the college town, I might die soon.

And yet I sat cross-legged on the patio table and felt the Presence of the "most High" *with* me . . . and in that "secret place," I knew I was safe . . . in triumph . . . in disaster . . . in laughter . . . in heartbreak . . . in sickness . . . in health . . . "Because Christ dwells in me, the ground on which I stand is holy ground because He is standing on it too."

I wrote in my journal:

I have found "the secret place of the most High" and I abide in it moment by moment. I believe it! I shall prove it! In whatever the future holds!

It came in a lightning flash of illumination and I knew. I accepted it and did not doubt. I was serene.

It was set as if I had been twiddling a radio knob and getting garbled sounds, and then, bang!, the sounds converged and clarified and the meaning emerged.

As I write these words, I am not anxious. I know little of the mystery of life, but I do know "the secret place of the most High." And I determine that in my "little boat," in my personal journey in "the dark, fearful gulf," I shall prove Him Truth.

7
Life's Greatest Mystery

When I was sixteen, the words of Psalm 91:1 enveloped my whole future in the assurance that I had a guarantee against trouble, disillusionment, and certainly faulty pituitary glands!

I had good reason to believe that.

I had read books that "proved" it . . .

I listened to personal testaments to it . . .

I heard sermons preached . . .

I remember well the imagery of one minister who filled my father's pulpit in a revival series. He had a son fighting at that time in World War II. I can still remember the intensity of his face, the pathos in his voice, the fervency of his belief as he stated: "My boy is safe wherever he is because my prayers assure that he is daily protected by 'the shadow of the Almighty.'"

His voice would drop lower. He would lean across the pulpit. His face would flame with devotion as he whispered with dramatic urgency, "And there is no bullet, no torpedo, no bomb in the world that can penetrate that 'shadow.'"

I remember the thrill of awed delight that charged through my veins. How wonderful to be a Christian and be assured that nothing bad would ever happen!

Near the close of that revival, he received a telegram.

The telegram.

His son had been killed in action.

I shall never forget the ashen look of his face, the tremble of his hands, the total sag of his body. His life-carousel was burning and he could find no water brigade of Scriptures to put out the flames.

He did not conclude the revival services. He left immediately for his home. I always wondered what happened to his faith.

Now it was my turn . . .

Jill was an "inner-circle" friend.

She came from across the country to see me.

She listened to the account of the diagnosis, the damage done to the body in crisis, the prognosis of early death unless I could find another way to live. She jumped from the sofa in her anger. She paced the floor in agitation.

Then she whirled and pounded on the table.

"It's unfair! It isn't right! You cannot *ever* convince me that this is God's will!"

To my amazement, I heard myself say: "No. I won't even try."

She looked at me in disbelief. She had not expected that answer.

She pounded on the table again and said: "I mean it, Ruth! This doesn't make any sense and so you are bound to be healed. Soon. We just have to *believe* that."

We studied each other in silence. I was surprised at my sudden sense of calm.

"Ruth, you *have* to demand a miracle! Because this isn't right! God didn't cause this."

I took a deep breath and slowly began to articulate some concepts that had been slow in coming. Born in the crucible of my soul's deepest agony, they had been incubating in heavelling frustration until they had matured enough for me to try to put them into words.

With an increasing confidence, I said: "Jill, I do not believe that God *causes* either joy or sorrow, health or suffering, clarity or frustration . . .

"I believe . . . that God is with us in all of life, working in the triumphs and the tragedies . . . Not *causing* them, Jill, but *using* them creatively . . . when we allow."

She looked at me in bewilderment.

"I have no earthly idea what you just said."

I grinned and nodded.

It was still new to me too. I was glad she was there to help me think.

I picked up the Bible. It opened easily to Psalm 91. I read the first verse.

"He that dwelleth in the secret place of the most High shall abide under the shadow of the Almighty."

Jill ran over to grab my hand.

"Ruth, don't you see that is the promise that makes me say you will be healed! I know you. Surely, of all the people I have observed closely, you're protected 'under the shadow of the Almighty.'"

"You mean that phrase is a guarantee of a life of bliss?" I asked her.

She paused.

"Well, I wouldn't say *that* . . . but . . ."

"But that is what you believe. That is what I've believed too. Until now. But as I've wrestled with this thing, I have had to understand that there are some things that God can*not* do!"

She swallowed hard. She could not believe her ears.

"You mean . . . you believe that God can*not* heal you?"

"I didn't say that."

I pulled her down beside me.

"Look, God created a world of natural law. Right?

"He has the power to break those laws . . . and He does indeed break them at times . . . but He is not obligated to do so. We live in a world of natural law. For the most part, God limits His power and allows us to live in natural law with all the resulting consequences. And He is always *with* us."

We sat silently together, hand-holding.

Redefining faith is terrifying, torturous.

Suddenly I remembered.

Thomas Costain had written an account in *The Silver Chalice* that had given me an important shaft of light. I went to the library and pulled the book from its shelf.

I leafed through it to a marked page and read aloud.

At this point in the book, Peter had met in the catacombs with a group of Christians who were deeply concerned because of Nero's promised execution of one hundred Christians on the next day. As the people gathered about their church leader, these are the words Peter spoke:

> This is in all of your minds . . . You are asking, 'Is it the will of God that these hundred men and women, all of whom believe in Jesus and strive to walk in His steps, shall be put to death for a crime of which they are innocent?' You are thinking, 'Surely the Hand of the Lord will be stretched out to save them.'

"You must remember," I reminded Jill, "that the Peter who was speaking was the same Peter who had been chained and guarded by *four* quaternions of soldiers in Herod Agrippa's jail. By a divine miracle of intervention in natural law, he was set free and walked out of incarceration.

"This was the same Peter who had walked on water, healed the sick, raised the dead.

"This man knew, as few have experientially known, the power of the Almighty to intervene in the consequences of natural law or free choice. But, in the story by Costain, he looked at the Christians huddled about him in the secrecy of the catacombs and said:

> My brethren . . . I can give you no answer save the one you have already heard. The Lord has not said 'Arise, Peter, and save them.' And truly, brothers and sisters in the faith, should we expect Him to speak? Listen, listen in patience and understanding. It is always known on the eve of a great battle that on the day following, thousands of fine young men will be cut down ruthlessly. Does the Lord feel it incumbent on Him to interfere in these tragic butcheries? When the forces of nature gather for the flooding of a mighty river or there is an agitation in the bowels of the earth and it is known in heaven that an earthquake will follow, the Lord does not reach down to remove the people who stand in the path of destruction. When a pestilence begins in the slums of a city, the Lord does not intervene to save the thousands who will die miserably of the plague. Life on this earth is made

cruel by the barbarities of nature and the wickedness of men, and thus it has been from the beginning.

Jill and I looked at each other searchingly.

What, then, was the meaning of the declarative statement that "He that dwelleth in the secret place of the most High shall abide under the shadow of the Almighty"? If the "shadow of the Almighty" were not a guarantee against the evils of natural law or of free choice of humanity . . . *what did it mean?*

After a time, I went to the library and pulled out another book. It was Hannah Whitall Smith's *The Christian's Secret of a Happy Life*. I turned to a page where a section was marked in red. I had read it over and over years ago. I had not understood.

Now, in a flash, I remembered . . . and so I read aloud to Jill the description given by a woman in a prayer meeting of an important spiritual experience. She had been in great pain because the free choices of other people in her world seemed to be destroying the beauty of God's handiwork.

Why God would permit such tragedy when He had the omnipotent power to prevent it was a question she could not resolve.

Until the moment when she had an interior vision.

Mrs. Smith tells of her account:

She thought she was in a perfectly dark place, and that there advanced toward her, from a distance, a body of light which gradually surrounded and enveloped her and everything around her. As it approached, a voice seemed to say, 'This is the Presence of God! This is the Presence of God!' While surrounded with this presence, all the great and awful things in life seemed to pass before her—fighting armies, wicked men, raging beasts, storms and pestilences, sin and suffering of every kind.

She shrank back at first in terror; but soon she saw that the Presence of God so surrounded and enveloped herself and each one of those things that not a lion could reach out its paw, nor a bullet fly through the air, except as the Presence of God moved out of the way to permit it.

And she saw that if there were so thin a film, as it were, of this glorious Presence between herself and the most terrible violence, not a hair of her head could be ruffled, nor anything touch her, except as the Presence decided to let the evil through. Then all the small and annoying things of life passed before her; and equally she saw that there also she was so enveloped in this Presence of God that not a cross look, nor a harsh word, not petty trial of any kind could affect her, unless God's encircling Presence moved out of the way to let it.

Jill reached for the book.

She studied the underlined words.

When she looked up, there were tears in her eyes.

"Shadow of the Almighty?" she asked.

I nodded.

"He is always with us . . . and 'the shadow of the Almighty' protects us from all consequences of natural law *or* free choice which would be irredeemable in His plans. But those things which *can* be redeemed for good . . . are allowed to progress with cause and effect."

Jill picked up Costain's book and we considered together.

When Peter was thrown in prison by Herod Agrippa, the resulting impoverishment of his leadership of the fledgling Christian faith was not redeemable *at that time*. The shadow of the Almighty intervened. Peter walked out of bonds and a guarded jail by divine miracle. Natural law and Herod Agrippa's free choice were circumvented by God.

But at the time of which Costain was writing, the baby church had grown from a few in one nation to thousands in many nations. At this time, the death of the one hundred Christians by Nero's crazed edict was redeemable. Perhaps even more illuminating, is that Peter's own imprisonment by Nero *at a later date* was redeemable.

Nero, as Herod, had Peter jailed under heavy guard. From that cell, he was led to his death. Neither natural law *nor* Nero's free choice were touched.

"The shadow of the Almighty" protected Peter from Herod Agrippa's jail and death edict. Nothing, No One protected Peter from Nero's jail and death edict.

"Perhaps, Jill," I mused, "the promise of Psalm 91:1 that we felt was a guarantee for the Christian that 'God's in His heaven; all's right *with the world*' . . . is, in reality, a guarantee that

'God's in His heaven; all's right *for His child*' . . . through His redemption."

She nodded slowly.

We sat together in the gathering duskiness of the den, silently letting new insights unseat old misconceptions and begin to relieve the hopelessness of our situation.

All of a sudden . . . WHAM! . . . it hit me!

I jumped to my feet, my face glowing, and I said: "Jill, listen! The 'shadow of the Almighty' is a promise of a sentence I wrote long ago and am only now beginning to comprehend.

"Remember when I was in the hospital in Kansas City, I wrote: 'Because He is a Redeemer God, He will enable me to make creative *use* of all, even unpleasant, circumstances?

"Jill, I had no idea then how *unpleasant* circumstances could be. I'm beginning to get a glimmer now.

"And so I have been cowering in fear, despairing in disillusionment, even scoffing at this promise as untruth . . . but Jill . . .

"*That* is what it means to 'abide under the shadow of the Almighty! *That* is what it means!"

I paced the floor in excitement as I tried to sort out my tumbling thoughts.

"To abide under the 'shadow of the Almighty' is to live free from fear of irredeemable circumstances! Although problems, frustrations, tragedies enter our lives, we know that not one of them is beyond 'working together for good' OR 'shadow of the Almighty' would have deterred it.

"So . . . we can know that on whatever 'ground' we find ourselves, He will be *with* us . . . and, if we allow, He will ultimately, in His time, in His way, redeem every tear, every anguish, every sorrow."

When Christ dwells in me, then the ground on which I stand is holy ground because He is standing on it too. And because He is a Redeemer God, He will enable me to make creative use of all, even unpleasant, circumstances.

In the spidery scrawl on the flyleaf of my Bible, I could now find answers for my torture points.

I had screamed before my burning life-carousel: *Who* is the most High? Answer: He is a Redeemer God. Redeemer of sin. Redeemer of circumstance.

I had shouted at the dancing flames of my life-dreams: "What is the secret place of the most High?" Answer: On whatever "ground I stand" . . . whatever changing scene it may be . . . He is *with* me.

I had bowed in agony as I gasped: "What does it mean 'to abide under the shadow of the Almighty'?" Answer: It means to "abide" with the knowledge that no problem, no frustration, no tragedy that enters our lives is irredeemable. He *will* enable us to make "creative *use* of all, even unpleasant, circumstances."

I do not say . . . oh, no! I do not say . . . that we who find life-suffering are blessed in our affliction. Yet I do assert that one can dimly see and humbly know that "life's greatest mystery" can be high adventure.

I am not, here, saying that old Puritan truism that "suffering teaches." I do not believe that, else all the world would be wise since everyone suffers physically, emotionally, mentally, one or all. But to deep pain *can* be added an openness of spirit so that one does learn vital clues that aid in comprehending suffering and assist in putting it into an understandable perspective that makes its ravages bearable—even, in a certain sense, filled with wonder.

William Blake said that "man was made for joy and woe" and that, once grasped, "through the world we safely go."

"He that dwelleth in the secret place of the most High shall abide under the shadow of the Almighty."

To make that assertion standing before a cross, itself signifying the suffering of God in the person of man and the redemption of man in the person of God illuminates mystery so that one's mind can go on to ponder the incredible paradox that the greatest sorrow and the greatest joy coexist on Golgotha.

8

A Sanctuary Lost

I can understand now, I think, why men seek their "moment of truth" in the bullring. Why they risk death on unconquered mountains . . . and in speeding cars.

It is that stripped-down insight they are seeking, when all the nonessentials fall away and only the core is left, only the reality of what life is all about!

It's a terrible thing. It's a wonderful thing . . . that moment . . . and, afterward, nothing can ever be the same again.

I know.

I didn't seek it in a bullring . . . or on a mountain . . . or in a racing car. In fact . . . I did not seek it at all.

It came all unexpected, all unwanted, all uninvited. But it did come . . . and nothing can ever be the same again.

I watched, with stricken streaming eyes, as years of academic expertise, years of experiential expertise equipping me for a myriad of fulfilling careers all whirled away in the smoke rings of my burning life-carousel.

Gasping in shock, shrieking in anger, sobbing in despair, I grabbed my beloved Psalm 91 and clutched its words for help.

Its first verse proved to be concepts God-given years before in my first glimpse of this dark spot on my life-horizon. And my returning faith was steadying, holding, comforting to my conscious mind. But in my subconscious, in my emotions . . . my

79

spirit was reeling, resisting, roaring denial.

My intellect could explore definitions in Psalm 91:1. Fine. It was an intellectual exercise.

But no matter how much logic I discovered, no matter how many new insights I perceived, no matter how much my *mind* accepted, that was *not* the area where pain was shredding spirit-slivers. In the *inner being*, intellectual comfort was disdained; it was even contemptible as I huddled before the dazzling consuming fires of *everything* I had expected life to be for me.

The mental understandings were splendid and high-sounding. My brain reached for acceptance . . . but my hurting heart demanded more.

I wrote in my journal at a time I was reading Eugenia Price:

"Redeemer God. Creative USE of tragedy.
God's way. God's time."
I know, Eugenia Price! I know!
I've studied it. I've reached for it. I've determined to prove it.
But I hurt, Genie! I'm throbbing with a passion that shatters my insides, wounds my body, and leaves me gasping.

It is all very well to look at toppled, cherished carousels, pick up burned, tortured pieces and talk of creative use. It is . . . words. Isn't it?

I remember Antigone's words, "I never knew how great the loss could be, even of sadness." One cannot know until the loss. And then, when it is so much greater than one ever dreamed, how does one go beyond talk . . . and find a way to build amid the rubble that remains?

It is all very well to quote Psalm 91:1 and believe that "He that dwelleth in the secret place of the most High shall abide under the shadow of Almighty" assures me of redemption of all, even unpleasant, circumstances. Somehow. Someway. Sometime.

But what about now? Sophocles said: 'To be wise is to suffer'. I qualify, but I am not wise! I can think logically, but, in reality, my heart has no notion what those mental processes mean!

It's kinda like discussing the pituitary gland with the doctors after diagnosis. It was mind-stretching and exciting. It had nothing to do with the way I lived my life.

I can think through Psalm 91:1 and find the promise of redemption of unpleasant circumstance. It is mind-stretching and exciting. It has nothing to do with the way I want to live my life!

But it does. It does.

Don't fight a fact, Ruth.

Deal with it.

But I don't know how!

And so I put the journal on the floor, curled my knees up to my breasts, and sobbed myself to sleep.

When I awoke, my body was stiff and my mood still vibrated with disillusion. I picked up my Bible and read Psalm 91:2: "I will say of the Lord, He is my refuge . . ."

I stared at the words. I was stunned that the psalmist had the effrontery to make such an assertion. And yet there it was in black and white.

And I had believed it for a lifetime!

Now I muttered: "Has *every* shred of my faith been childish optimism?"

I had moments when I gained a toehold on the mountain of faith, but only moments. For my toes seemed to always root in shale that quickly gave way and I dropped into the abyss below.

I had moments of rational thought where my intellect could force the quiet of my spirit . . . but only moments. For the child emotions of a heart that was observing the total dissolution of everything I had planned for, prepared for, and was experiencing could *not* be quelled with adult concepts. My entire understanding of *life* was founded in activity, performance, giving. My entire understanding of *God* was founded in service.

So, as the doctor's words reeled through my mind: *Never be active; never perform; never give* (as I translated the word) . . . all my understandings of life dissolved.

Never be of God-service (as I defined the term) . . . all my understandings of *God* were sucked into the quicksand of total frustration.

I read Psalm 91:2 and cried.

Obediently, happily, with total childlike trust, I had said those words for a lifetime. Now, in spite of my adult understanding of Psalm 91:1, I found that I was totally incapable of saying the words of Psalm 91:2 with an iota of honesty.

I could *say* them.

I did not *mean* them.

How could I?

Refuge? Refuge?

If the Lord is my refuge, then what had happened to all the virtues of refuge: Protectiveness. Peace. Prosperity.

My mind could assert that He is a Redeemer God who is *with* me and who will not allow anything to enter my life that is *irredeemable*, but my heart could not tolerate going on to say: *He is a refuge!*

No. Not that!

Refuge would have prevented all this.

Did that give the lie to my intellectually-accepted concept that nothing would enter my life that *was* irredeemable?

I could only hold my head in tormented frustration and sob.

Was Truth falsehood?

Was Black white?

Was Up down?

My mind clung to something solid in Psalm 91:1. There was an imperturbable solidity there, a kind of flinty certainty that held . . . even as my heart shrieked in total denial of Psalm 91:2: "I will say of the Lord, He is my refuge . . ."

No. No.

Redeemer God . . . enable me to make creative use of all, even unpleasant, circumstance . . . all of that seemed acceptable to my mind, but it was a *long* way off in the future. Sometime . . . Somewhere . . . there might be redemption. There might be a new world. There might be creative *use of . . .* Yes . . . I could accept that.

For the future.

But refuge was in the present. And that simply was *not* reality.

Explain Yourself, again I pleaded with God. *Explain how I could have any reason to now assert You are my refuge! Look! Look at my life! There is no refuge here! . . . O God, why? O my dear God, why?*

Lines from some poet responded:

Distressed mind, forbear to tease the hooded why.
The shape will not reply.

And again my sarcasm shrilled in harshness.

*Why won't You reply? Are You caught in cosmic embarrass-
ment? I have spent my whole life preparing to be of service to You!
And here I have been: Giving lavishly of my time, my talent, my
energies, my expertise, my laughter, my love . . . All I asked from
You was refuge . . . a healthy body which would allow such God
service! This isn't a self-made mess . . . but Yours!*

*No! I have some theological assertions that I will say of the Lord.
But I cannot say: He is my refuge!*

And I closed my journal and sobbed in anguish.
I knew an era in my life was over.
I knew a sanctuary had been lost.
And then one afternoon, my collegiate son, Billy, came to
our house. He was a school bus driver and he parked the yellow
monster in front. He paused to tease Ron in the den; then came
to the bedroom where I lay in my pea-green limpness.

He leaned against the dresser and said: "I just wanted to
come by and tell you where I am in my thinking."

My eyes filled with tears.

I knew the intensity of his suffering with me. No refuge for
me. No refuge for Billy.

Ever-heart-close to me, he had gone through the long slide
into diagnosis with me. He had listened, observed, held my
hand. And he had jumped in the excitement of my returning
health after replacement therapy.

The exuberant essence of *I* was returned and life was *good*
again.

And then . . . so quickly . . . came crisis.

Bill told me of the look on Billy's face when they lifted my
unconscious body into the ambulance plane to fly me back to the
team of endocrine specialists who had made the diagnosis. Could
their expertise save me now?

My son had watched the plane taxi away that day and he
knew, with deep certainty, that he might never see his mother
alive again.

Although death was averted, the harsh prognosis, the de-cree to leave our known world had augmented Billy's suffering. As he leaned against the dresser, my mother-heart rushed out to envelop him in a protective blanket that would, somehow, take away the pain.

But when I looked into his brown eyes, I knew I could not do that. The wound was deep. The intensity of soul-agony was etched on his face. Pain hauntingly hunched his shoulders.

I looked at my beautiful son and took a shuddering breath.

My life-carousel was burning.

So was Billy's.

I could douse neither.

Refuge! my heart cried . . . *O God, why haven't You been a refuge?*

Slowly my mind turned outward to listen to his husky voice. His words were startling.

"You know I've always loved God, been a Christian . . . and all that," he said. "But I just floated along in it. Never thought much about it really. When we got into bull sessions in the dorm about whether or not we believed the Bible, the virgin birth, the reality of the Christian faith, I could get into the discussion in wide dimensions, letting doubt push, pull, even, for moments, convince."

His hands in his pockets, he straightened his shoulders and looked at me keenly.

"And then this happened . . . I watched you and Daddy carefully through all of the events. Ron told me that he was at the kitchen table when that firm called from Washington D.C. and offered Daddy $35,000 to come there in public relations. He thanked them and turned them down on the spot.

"When he hung up, Ron said, 'Daddy, why did you do that? You don't know where you are going next year. Why didn't you at least hold them for a while?'

"Ron said that Daddy just grinned and said: 'I don't know where the Lord is leading us next year, but I doubt that four academic degrees and thirteen years in the ministry have been preparing me for public relations.'

"And that was that.

"When Ron told me, we both looked at each other soberly. We had always known he was a strong man. His trust in that one moment made him a giant. We knew how privileged we were to be witnesses.

"So . . . now as I pray and meditate, I have begun to really comprehend what Christianity is all about. It isn't just a theory to toss around in dorm bull sessions. It isn't just a ritual to go through on Sunday and in family prayer. It isn't just a doctrine, a creed. As I've watched you and Daddy in all this, I've seen so clearly that Christianity is a Personality that will hold you rock steady *when all the chips are down.*"

The tears flooded and I gasped for breath. My heart was bulging with so much gratitude and pride that I thought I truly might suffocate.

His voice had been soft and threaded with deep feelings. He leaned over and rumpled my hair. And then to shatter the emotion-charged moment, he straightened and spoke briskly and with determination.

"Out of all this trauma has emerged my faith. And as I clasp it to me, I feel an increasing 'sense of oughtness' that I should let go my plans for law school and structure new ones to enter the ministry."

I choked on a sob.

I could hardly believe my ears.

All his life Billy had planned to be a lawyer. He had read everything on Clarence Darrow, written research papers on the famous lawyer's persuasion techniques, and majored in communication with the goal of emulating Darrow in criminal law. He had never, once, mentioned even a passing interest in church work.

I wiped my eyes to better see him. I shook my head to be certain my hearing wasn't affected.

He was still talking, his words tumbling over each other as he sorted out his thoughts.

"Now that I personally know the reality of Christianity when all the chips are down, I feel a compulsion to spend my life sharing that truth . . . especially with youth. I think, maybe, God is leading me into youth ministry . . ."

I was even more stunned.

His beloved father was a minister, so he could conceivably want to emulate him. But this was not emulation. This was response to a personally-called, personally-unique ministry for God . . . and I wondered why, after all these years of deafness to such a possibility . . .

And then an insight was born: *Billy had never been hurt before!*

He had grown up in a warm cocoon of love that truly had been a refuge from anything unpleasant. His school career had been successful socially, athletically, academically. He had enjoyed uninterrupted good fortune.

It was only in the moment when all that was stripped away from him, when "all the chips were down," to use his phrase, that he had sought and found God for himself. Until he was flung into our family crucible of suffering, Billy had floated along in sterility and banality of faith.

I turned back into his stream of speech.

"You know the record we had as children? The one about the little engine that struggled up the hill because it was so determined?

I think I can.

I think I can.

I think I can . . . and then it reached the top!

"Well, I think that sorta was my philosophy of life. Until now. If things got a bit tough, I'd just grit my teeth and mutter:

I think I can.

I believe I can.

I'm sure I can . . . and I always could.

"I was competent on my own . . ." He paused. "I never needed God."

He rubbed his hand across his face.

"But in all of this, I splattered right into impossibility. I could repeat the brave little engine's ditty till I was hoarse. It didn't change one thing. My mother was still very ill. My parents were still going to move away. My mother still might die."

His lashes were tangled with tears.

"And then I needed God. And when I cried to Him, He

came to me. I knew that He was *real."* His voice was choking again, but he jauntily tossed off the emotion and said: "So! I thought I would stop by and just let you know where my thoughts are these days. Nothing definite yet. But I'm working on it."

His lips brushed my cheek.

"I'll keep you informed," he said. And he was gone.

I lay very still . . . my emotions rioting, my mind still stunned.

"Truth pierces matter where the heart is rent," I quoted softly. And, for the first time, I understood that phrase.

Billy had lived twenty years in the refuge of perennial bliss. He had not needed or found God for himself.

But now, in months of intense helplessness and chaos, he had discovered his need and discovered his God . . . and, perhaps, he had discovered a new life-career.

The intensity of my thoughts made me sit up.

Yes. I could see it. God's wisdom was so much better than mother-love.

Were I to have my way, Billy would never know the sting of tears.

But the all-wise Redeemer God "stepped aside" and allowed the dragons of incurable illness, of life-changing edicts, of closeness to death for a loved one to smack pandemonium into the serenity of my son's life.

The dissolution of his peace was now the source of his *becoming.*

I grabbed my robe and headed for the den. It seemed I could think better in there. I was beginning to feel a shift in my understanding. I slipped onto the sofa and drew my knees under my chin.

"I will say of the Lord: He is my refuge . . ."

I bit my lip in study.

That I was wrong in my earlier definition was established. Now I was beginning to get a batwing of a new perception . . . one that included all kinds of unpleasant circumstances. The Lord was not a "refuge" against adversity. Ah no! He is much wiser than that.

I shook my head in incredulity.

My mother-love for Billy was a "refuge" in the sense that I had defined it.

But Mother-love coddled.

Mother-love babied.

Mother-love hedged out growth.

Hey! Was that true? Could spiritual retardation be due to snuggling in the "refuge" of not facing reality . . . not looking squarely at life as it really is?

Oh, I would have spared Billy all this unhappiness.

But as I had listened to him, my heart had soared on a crescendo of praise because I could feel, see, hear his *using* the pain to expand, mature, grow up.

I sat in the den that day and, for the first time, understood that God is my "refuge" . . . not in the sense of my warm human security . . . but in the sense that whatever the Redeemer God permits to enter my life, He will enable me to use creatively. Now *that* is "refuge!" Not refuge from learning, or from growing, or from advancing, even through pain . . . but "refuge" from waste, from immobility, from stagnation.

How impoverished would be Billy's life if my love were his "refuge." No. I could see that Billy needed the *coup de grace*, the wound of mercy, to make him totally unhappy, totally insecure, totally helpless. Only then could he shrug off the complacency and comforts of childhood and take necessary strides toward becoming a man. Only then could he discover his personal need and claim God as his *own* reality.

So.

"Refuge." How to define it after these insights?

Mr. Webster said refuge is a "place of protection." Protection. Against what?

My heart did a flip-flop of comprehension.

Refuge: A place of protection against defeat.

When Christ dwells in me, then the ground on which I stand is holy ground because He is standing on it too. And because He is a Redeemer God, He will enable me to make creative USE of all, even unpleasant, circumstances.

Yes.

I understood.

Finally.

"I will say of the Lord: He is my refuge . . ." not in the sense of protection from life's ills, but in the sense that we have a bonded *guarantee against defeat* . . . in whatever season we come!

I wrote in my journal:

There has to come a day when I find a way to build for the second half of my life much as I built for the first: creatively, with my whole heart. It is God's way not to WASTE anything. Even sorrow. Even suffering. Even burned carousels. So there will be a way for me to do something beyond enduring the severed stump of my life, something beyond accepting the mere comfort of God's Presence, something beyond the solace of rest in a "limited" body.

I am convinced that He is a Redeemer of circumstance, as well as of sin. He will not waste this illness if I give Him a chance to redeem it. I must remain open . . .

I am going to go on.

God does not punish by illness or broken life-plans. I settled that long ago. If He does, then Jesus Christ did not reveal Him rightly. Jesus entered into human suffering. He did not remain aloof from it. So I am now waiting, as openly as I know how, for Him to show me how He is going to make USE of my dead carousel. I must not waste any of it.

Refuge. I see it now. I wonder that I did not before. It means that I trust God the way I trusted my daddy. That is a finite example but it is one that I best understand. Daddy's love for me did not make my life free of suffering, but he was always caring, supporting, assisting in healing, in rebuilding, in finding creative use of.

Refuge. God does not protect me from pain or joy. God does not cause either pain or joy. God works in and through the tragedies and happinesses of the haphazard of earthly life, making redemptive use of . . . everything. I am protected from waste, for this is what "I will say of the Lord: He is my refuge . . ."

At this writing, Billy, now a college graduate, is in the full-time youth ministry. He often exults at how superior is this life-work for the fulfillment of the uniqueness of himself than law school would have been. Ah yes! Creative *use* of pain for Billy. God did prove Himself a "refuge" for Billy.

Not in Mother-protecting terms.
But in God-*redeeming* facts.
Life can bring grief.
Life can*not* bring failure when God is our *refuge!*

9

I Never Knew
a Heart Could Hurt
So Much!

I was not afraid of death.

I was convinced of immortality.

Threescore years and ten of "measuring out our life with coffee spoons," as T. S. Eliot phrased it, was illogical. If it were, it would be too pointless, too tedious a game for participant and spectator alike, too banal a drama for so spectacular a set. But more, Jesus proved immortality. I believed it.

To love life, then, is to love death because death is life's fulfillment. Death is only the door into the larger life.

It was not fear of death that was my torture point.

It was my fear of life "in limited parameters." And, try as I would, I could not seem to get beyond it.

I understood that loving life is accepting its rhythms and moving in step with them; subordinating ambitions and pursuits to the natural ebb and flow rather than striving, like King Canute, to impose one's own authority. But I was paralyzed with a cement cast of terror that held me immobile. I was caged in a prison of guilt whose origin or dimensions I could not understand.

Emily Dickinson phrased it:

> Of God we ask one favor,
> That we may be forgiven—
> For what, He is presumed to know—

91

> The Crime, from us, is hidden—
> Immured the whole of Life—
> Within a magic Prison
> We reprimand the Happiness
> That too competes with Heaven.

Yes. Somehow the torture point had to do with "hidden crime" . . . a child's plea for forgiveness . . . but I could not understand.

I truly did not believe that God punished by illness, death, personal tragedy. I did not accept my severed-life-stump as divine chastisement.

And yet the torture point remained.

Since I could not think it through, I went back to Psalm 91:2. "I will say of the Lord, He is my refuge and my fortress . . ."

At sixteen, I had blithely believed *fortress* to be synonymous with *refuge*, both of which were defined as protection from unpleasantness. Now I turned to the dictionary to discover the meaning of the separate word, *fortress*.

Mr. Webster defines *fortress* as a "fortified place with troops, guns, etc." A second explanation is "a military post."

I shook my head in total bewilderment.

It made no sense.

Strain the brain machine in my cranium as I would, I could not find meaning in the phrase: "I will say of the Lord, He is my *military post fortified with troops, guns, etc.*"

I let it go until one afternoon when I was perusing the journal account of my meditations of the Lord as "refuge." I was suddenly startled by a new insight.

My entire understanding of life was founded in activity, performance, giving. . . . My entire understanding of God was founded in *service* . . . so as a doctor's words reeled through my mind: *Never be active; perform; give* (as I translated the term) . . . all my understandings of God were sucked into the quicksand of total frustration.

And in that frustration, I had lashed out at God for not being my refuge. Now . . . as I carefully considered . . . I knew that it was not anger against God . . . it was anger . . . against *me!*

The equation I had built my definition of life upon . . . the equation I had built my concept of God upon . . . was:

Performance = Goodness
Non-Performance = Badness

And . . . performance . . . was intrinsically linked with health!

I remembered the long line of hospital rooms in which I had been placed prior to diagnosis. In each of them, I could remember my tears, my strain, my utter sincerity as I promised God over and over that if I could be released, I would be "good" and *do* all the things I was supposed to do . . . to be worthy of Life, to be of *service* to God.

How deeply earnest were my vows that I wouldn't be "bad" (translation: *ill*) any more! Only God can know how intensely I promised I would perform!

So, when released, I dashed back into all my responsibilities, lavishly burning all my energies. To my dismay, the illness would clutch my body, and once again I would be returned to the hospital, proof that I had *not* been "good" (translation: *healthy, performing*) . . . after all.

I had lied.

And I hated myself.

It was that same equation that had thrust me into crisis.

Following diagnosis, with the return of the zest for life, I was determined to be "good" forever! So when my body sagged, I gave stern self-lectures and raced on. Into death. And now the damage was such that God-service, as I understood it, was denied me.

I had been chewing on my pencil as I perused the words in my journal. As I comprehended these realities, I bit off the eraser in my gasping pain.

I spit the eraser out and stood to walk to the window.

No wonder I had cried.

No wonder I had screamed at God.

My previous life-concepts told my sincere child-heart that, in spite of all my adult intellectual discussions of the Redeemer

God, the "crime" remained: I was "bad," no longer worthy of life, no longer of value in God-service. And those intolerable facts marched like a batallion of heavy-booted, fully armed, strategically trained soldiers onto my life's battleground and their approach bulged my heart with abject terror.

I looked clearly, now, at my "crime" and observed that batallion of equations marching steadily, rhythmically, arrogantly to defeat all that remained of my life.

ONE, TWO, THREE, FOUR

ONE, TWO, THREE, FOUR

They marched with determined, destined, deadly tread.

ONE, TWO, THREE, FOUR

ONE, TWO, THREE, FOUR

I had been "bad"! As a result, my life was of no use to anyone.

As a result, there was no God-service left in me.

ONE, TWO, THREE, FOUR

ONE, TWO, THREE, FOUR

They were marching to overwhelmingly defeat all that remained of me.

I stood, knee-deep in "badness," and observed with quaking heart as those almighty, military equations marched to destroy me. And then . . . they halted abruptly, almost in midstep, and poised in immobility . . . waiting.

For what?

And then I "heard" the flaming words of my Lord, memorized long ago from their biblical record:

Thus saith the Lord that created thee, . . . and he that formed thee, . . . Fear not: for I have redeemed thee, I have called thee by thy name; thou art mine.

When thou passest through the waters, I will be with thee; and through the rivers, they shall not overflow thee: when thou walkest through the fire, thou shalt not be burned; neither shall the flame kindle upon thee.

For I am the Lord thy God, the holy one of Israel, thy Saviour.

Since thou wast *precious* in my sight, thou hast been *honourable*, and I have loved thee:

Fear not: for I am with thee.

(Isa. 43:1-5, *italics mine*)

Before my astonished eyes, the false equations turned heel and marched out of my sight.

I looked out the window at the wide expanse of green lawn, the redbird winging from shrub to shrub, and felt, as I think Moses must have felt when he stood before the burning bush . . . awed, humbled, grateful beyond articulation of words or thoughts.

The Lord that created me . . . He that formed me . . . considered me . . . not "bad" because illness had felled me, ceased my performing, burned my carousel . . . but the Lord considers me "honourable" and, in His Word, He says He loves me. He says I should never be afraid. For He is . . . I gasped in comprehension . . . He is my *fortress.*

He is like a military post fortified with troops and guns. He will put to rout any batallions that come to attack

Whether they march in ceaseless rows of false perceptions.

Whether they march in merciless lines of misunderstandings.

Whether they march in vicious formations of untrue equations.

Against *untruth,* I will say of the Lord: He is my Fortress!

"I am with thee," He says. "Thou art mine. I have *redeemed* thee. For I am the Lord thy God, the Holy One of Israel, thy Saviour . . ."

I went to my knees in worship as my mind was illumined with the knowledge that He is my Savior in the sense of salvation from sin. And . . . He is my Savior in the sense of salvation from devastating attack from the enemy.

The Lord is my Savior in the military sense of that term.

He has troops, weapons, ammunition that will ensure my safety from destruction so long as I am in His Presence . . . for He loves me.

Softly I whispered: *Thank You.* I was enveloped in a holy hush as the portrait of the Lord as my fortress began to sink deeply into the layers of my spirit, pushing out all lingering guilt of the "hidden crime," enveloping each tissue, each corpuscle in

His loving acceptance, for which forgiveness was unnecessary.

Later, I wrote in my journal:

Now that the batallion of False Equations:

Performance = Goodness
Non-Performance = Badness

has been soundly turned back by my Fortress, I find my heart filled with awed wonder and songs of praise. I remember that, in Old Testament times, when Pharaoh and his armies were astoundingly drowned in the Red Sea by divine miracle, Moses sang: "The Lord is a man of war: the Lord is his name" (Exod. 15:3). And his sister, Miriam, took a timbrel in her hand and led the women in a victory-dance of wonder and praise.

I don't have a timbrel.

I'm too weak to dance.

But my spirit rejoices in the image of Miriam . . . and in my heart I exult in that same catapulting victory. I sing with Moses: "The Lord is a man of war: the Lord is His Name." I sing with the psalmist: "I will say of the Lord, He is my fortress!"

In addition to Joy, there are Hope, Faith, Security.

Now I have the freedom,

the courage,

the faith to begin to build for the second period of my life much as I built for the first: with my whole heart, creatively. My "badness" did not destroy the world of activity. My "goodness" has nothing whatever to do with performance.

I wonder why I never knew that before.

But I didn't.

God knows how desperately I yearned and how much I enjoyed serving Him in dynamic activity. I believe He used *that* service to His glory.

But that isn't the only reason for my existence.

He did not create me to *perform* for Him.

He created me as His child . . . to love me, to find me "precious," to call me "honourable" as I faced life *with* Him.

He created me to *be with* Him. *Doing* is no challenge for the

Creator-God who made this incredible universe. He had no need of my human efforts to keep His world in operation, His church alive and well.

I grinned in embarrassment.

What a ridiculous value I had placed on my efforts to perform.

I understood why.

That is where the dazzle lay.

That is what brought the gold trophies and awards.

That is what invited human compliments.

And that was all nice, but . . . *God* was not dazzled!

God had smiled in indulgent Fatherly pride at my honors—in the same way I had smiled when Billy and Ronnie won baseball trophies . . . nice, but nothing to do with *their* value!

God did not place value on exterior sparkle. The words in Isaiah 43 said that He loved, honored, found *me* precious. Just . . . *me.* Simple. Quiet. Unastounding . . . me.

God had created me to be.

When doing was a part of my life, He could and would use it for His glory. But when doing was no longer possible (in the sense that I defined that term), He was not panicked. He considered it no "crime." For the doing was the "lesser part" of God-service. Of course! He had told Martha that. (See Luke 10:42.) It was the *being* that was vital.

I scrawled across a page:

I intend to trust God's love for me. I will move through every change in my life, happy or sad, depending on the fact that God knows me as I really am . . . and loves me. He finds me "precious."

I cannot write those words without falling tears. My certainty of the "hidden crime" of badness has been such a torture point that now it has been removed, my whole being sobs with relief and gladness.

For I was always full of guilt. It went on all the time, without my realizing it. The knowledge that I was BAD shivered through my head just the way it had shivered through my head five minutes earlier. It reeled round and round. I couldn't catch it, couldn't catch it, couldn't catch it . . .

As I look back, I understand the intensity of my responses. The pain ripped every fiber. I never knew a heart could hurt so much! Although my carousel still lies in ruins, I can now have the freedom to truly dare to allow God to make redemptive use of my entire life: the tragedies as well as the triumphs; the tears as well as the smiles.

I doubt that I will ever find out the intellectual particulars my mind would like in regard to God's answer to human sorrow. But I believe faith is being a child with God. The only answer I truly know about life is living with God in the same kind of total trust a child wants to place in his father.

I will find a way to go on. Even now.

I promise.

10

A New Notebook

When the world was turning spring, I bought a new notebook. It was red with a picture of a bluebird in its center.

I held it to my nose to smell the ink, the alluring aroma a new notebook always gave me. It made me tingle with anticipation for the hours of page-filling.

Since I was working with Psalm 91, I supposed that should be my place to begin again. So I wrote across the top of page one: Psalm 91:3: "Surely he shall deliver thee from the snare of the fowler . . ."

As in the other verses, my mind was boggled by previous understandings. I couldn't seem to get beyond it.

In desperation, I went to the dictionary to reaffirm my definition of the terms. I found that I was correct in the assumption that a snare is a steel trap used by the "fowler" or hunter in search of wild birds. Although its design varies widely, its purpose is always the same: imprisonment of the winged creature.

I did understand the key words.

But the meaning of the verse eluded me.

Years earlier, my sixteen-year-old mind had fastened on the definition that I, the winged creature, would never be imprisoned by unpleasant circumstance. I starkly confronted that untruth and . . . in the declarative statement in Psalm 91:3, I could find no other meaning.

"Surely he shall deliver thee from the snare of the fowler . . ."

I wearily dropped the new notebook on the coffee table, wishing I had stopped with the breakthrough on verse two. I went out and lay in the sun.

Later a friend joined me.

Her chatter poured over my troubled mind like soothing syrup. I paid little attention to content until I heard her say: "I could have spared him all this if he had listened . . . but he chose not to . . . and so now he's caught . . . and I just have to go through it with him."

I frowned.

Somehow her words seemed significant. I had no idea why.

"Kathy, would you repeat that?"

Her free-falling verbal flood poised for a moment of silence and then it fell. "What do you mean . . . repeat? Repeat *what?* I was telling you that Dave has refused this entire semester to work on that term paper. He maintained it was to be a personal evaluation. I took that course last semester and I *knew* it was to be a full-blown research paper. But would he listen? Not for a minute! You *know* how he is! He just ignored me . . . and so now he's trapped in his room studying like mad . . . and I, who could have spared him all this, will have to carry his meals to him, keep the children quiet, and sleep without him until he gets done in days what should have taken weeks . . ."

The amazing Niagara of verbiage tumbled on, but my mind had grabbed her concept. Kathy's husband, Dave, was a student at the college.

Enrolled in my husband's persuasion class, he had misinterpreted the assignment and had chosen to ignore his wife's warnings that the previous semester she had written a term paper. Now in the last days of the semester, he was confronted with the reality of a "full-blown research paper" soon due. And he had done no work.

So, according to Kathy, he was now "trapped in his room studying like mad."

"Trapped in his room studying like mad . . ." or "caught in the snare of the fowler"?

I shook my head, trying to clear it.

I felt an insight trembling just beyond my reach.

"Surely he shall deliver thee from the snare of the fowler"
. . . but to interpret that statement as immunity from entrapment was false. My life had proved that. So what, then?

Kathy's voice broke through my study.

"It was his fault. I told him that. He didn't listen to Dr. Vaughn's assignment. And he didn't listen to my warnings. So he got himself into this mess. And he will just have to pay the consequences." Her voice was suddenly filled with giggles. "And that means no basketball game tonight!"

What was it I was looking for?

What insight could be gained from Dave's dilemma?

"Surely he shall deliver thee from the snare of the fowler . . ." *Deliver thee . . .*

Hey! I had thought those words were a guarantee that I would never be *trapped* by unpleasant circumstances, but that would be ignoring man's free will. God could be yearning to guide me to another path away from the "snare of the fowler" . . . but if I *chose* to follow another path, I could get caught!

Just as Dave had in his classwork.

His wife had warned him for an entire semester that he was going to run into the "snare" of a "full-blown research paper." He had *chosen* to ignore her. Now he was "trapped" . . . "studying like mad" . . . "missing the basketball game" . . . because "he got himself into this mess. And he will just have to pay the consequences."

Now, although Dave had ignored Kathy's pleas, and had plunged into the "snare," she was still *with* him. And because she loved him, she would "just have to go through it with him." She would "deliver" him from the "snare" of the term paper. She would help him find deliverance from a failing grade by pitching in to meet the crush of the schedule.

Is God like that?

Does God strive to warn us of "snares" in our lives? But because He gives free will, allows us to plunge headlong into them . . . *if we choose!* And because He loves us, He will simply be *with* us as we struggle inside the "trap" and then sets about helping us find deliverance by pitching in to help pick up the pieces, bind up the wounds, and find a creative way to go from there!

Ah! I had not seen that before.

God would be denying my free choice if He grabbed me and *refused to allow* me to get myself in a mess! Instead He could warn me in many ways, but if I misunderstood or ignored His directives, I had the *right* to hurl myself in the "snare" if I chose.

Is that why the verse said "deliver" . . . not "protect"? God would protect, when possible. Or, He would deliver, bind up the wounds, and *redeem* . . . when allowed.

Kathy had stopped her endless word supply to take a bite of some chocolate cake. I seized the opportunity to try the new insight on her.

When I had finished explaining, she nodded thoughtfully.

"Yes. I see that. I think that's right. But how does that fit in your case? Pituitary failure wasn't a snare you could have avoided by listening to God . . ."

Not wanting to give up the conversational ball, she continued to reel out her ideas . . . "But we don't fall into all 'snares" because of our own bad choices. There are the times we are victims of others' choices. Like me. My parents divorced. That was a bad time for me. And my choice had nothing to do with it. So it was a 'snare' I had no control over. But I sure got trapped in it. Like you say, because God loved me, He helped me through the pain of it. He helped me heal. He helped me find ways to use the disaster of my parents' lives to strengthen my own commitment to marriage and motherhood. They sure showed me what *not* to do!"

Kathy is one of those fascinating individuals whose words cascade from her lips every moment she is not eating or sleeping.

Her mind and tongue sped onward.

"And then there's you. You got trapped inside that body. You met the 'snare' of natural law, just as people who are in the path of a tornado or in an earthquake or in a storm at sea are victims of natural law."

She stopped long enough to grin.

"Of course, in your case, it is two kinds of snares! You're imprisoned in the 'snare' of natural law . . . and you're also

trapped by your own choice to misunderstand the doctors' explanation of the illness and to ignore all the warnings of your body.
That crisis that damaged so devastatingly is . . ."

She paused . . . and to my total delight, I saw that she was
embarrassed.

To embarrass Kathy enough to cause her to stop talking is a
feat to be proud of. She had almost said that the crisis was *my*
fault . . . and although accusations of Dave's faulty ways danced
off her tongue, she was appalled at having almost accused *me*.

I laughed, grabbed her to me (cake and all!), and kissed her.

Because, of course, she was right.

And for the first time in my life, that verse had real meaning.

"Surely he shall deliver thee from the snare of the fowler
. . ." He would guide me around the "snare" of unpleasant circumstances,, when it was possible without His interfering with
natural law or with free choice (others' or mine). But when the
"snare" grabbed me as a consequence of natural law or free
choice, He would be *with* me. He would enable me to make
creative *use* of the pain. He would *deliver* me from the devastation of the "snare." He would not allow its fangs to fasten upon
me and harm me in any way that was irredeemable in His hands.

He did not promise I would not ever be imprisoned by
unpleasant circumstance. He did promise I would not be defeated
for He would *deliver* me.

After Kathy left, I rushed to grab the new notebook. I
wanted to put it all down: *Kathy, Dave, term papers, fowlers'
snares, natural law, free choice* . . . my fingers sped in the record-
ing. As I wrote the last words: *He did promise I would not be
defeated, for He would deliver me* . . . I experienced one of those
rare moments when the old world bends its hoary head, and I
held my breath as all of my being flowed into a vast acceptance. I
knew that in the acceptance was victory. I could not put it into
words but as I remained still, unmoving, hardly breathing, the
rim of the darkness of the future seemed to lift a little, a very
little, and I could see, feel, touch the warmth of God's smile.

I had looked deep inside myself and found Him there.
Nothing could ever take that from me.

Now that I was not interpreting Scripture from a background of clichés, truisms, and platitudes, I was focusing on the specifics of each word, asking for a clear-cut definition.

So when I went back to the new notebook, I carried with me the dictionary to discover that one of the definitions of *pestilent* was "anything annoying, troublesome." A definition of *pestilence* is "an epidemic."

I leaned back in my chair and grinned as I wrote the remainder of Psalm 91:3: "Surely he shall deliver thee from the snare of the fowler, and from the noisome pestilence."

The two were not synonymous. Nor was the last some vague figure of speech the psalmist had thrown in for good measure. It was distinct and important.

"He shall deliver me from epidemics of annoying, troublesome problems," I wrote. *Deliver.* Not protect from.

I understood.

I was, at that moment, being blistered by a sandstorm epidemic of annoying, troublesome problems. Bill had resigned his position at the college and accepted the position of associate pastor of a large church in Denver. We were preparing for the move.

With that epic decision finalized, life should all be serenity and bliss. Right?

Wrong.

We had a house. There seemed to be no buyers.

There was packing to be done. I had always been the expert packer. Not one of my three men had ever packed a box before. And I was having trouble lifting a handkerchief.

The windows needed to be washed; the carpets, shampooed; there seemed to be no help. The assertion "I don't do windows!" also included dirty carpets and all other problem areas of a full house's becoming empty.

Bill was busy directing an important play in which Billy had a major role. I saw them rarely.

Ron was morose at the thought of leaving his beloved world and my heart ached for him. He was debonair on the outside; inside, I knew his stomach was doing the elephant stomp!

I wrote in my new notebook this poem:

Ron doesn't care that life's upside down:
   What was clear is night;
   What was black is white;
   What was seen is out of sight.
The future leers before him like a wicked clown
But Ron doesn't mind that life's upside down
   But his stomach does!

And, of course, there were business decisions to be made about the house in Denver, arrangements of furniture, what would fit where . . . Whee! Landslide of catastrophe! Whirlwind of things "annoying, troublesome." I was deluged with "noisome pestilence" and my mood was often grim.

With this new insight, I repeated: "Surely he shall deliver thee . . . from the noisome pestilence." He shall deliver thee . . . but only . . . only . . . *if I permit.*

I was cowering now in the deluge of problems. That was my right, God-given. *If I chose that.*

But . . . He was standing at that moment ready to deliver me from the "noisome pestilence" . . . *if I chose.*

That brought me smack up against reality.

I am responsible for my moods.

I am responsible for my emotions.

I am not their victim. I like to say that I am. I like to say "This feeling came over me . . ." or "I can't help it, but I'm depressed, or angry, or afraid . . ." but those are untruths.

"This feeling" may come over me, but it is my choice as to what I do with it. I can welcome it with open arms and settle back to bask in self-pity and woe . . . or . . . I can choose to allow the Redeemer God to *deliver me.*

I may feel depression, anger, fear . . . but I *can* help it! It is my *choice* as to whether I shall be overcome by the annoying troubles of my life . . . or whether *I* shall overcome.

The choice is mine. My mental, emotional dial is in my hand.

Oh, wow! I wish it weren't! It would be so much easier to be a martyr. So much easier! I don't like the responsibility for my mental outlook.

I don't like it. But it is true.

Because although the "epidemic of annoying troubles" floods my life, the Redeemer God will *deliver* me . . . *only if I choose.*

I snuggled in my "noisome pestilence."

That sounds ridiculous, but it is reality. Although there is unhappiness in such a state, there is also something morbidly inviting about wallowing in all the specifics of *"Woe is me!"* And God, because he loves so incredibly, stands by permitting me to *choose* to wallow there.

I took a deep breath.

Redeemer God, I prayed aloud, *You know about the house that won't sell; the packing that won't pack itself; the windows and carpets covered with dirt; Bill's and Billy's absence; the agitation in Ron's spirit, the problems of the move. You know about all of that. Amazingly, as You engineer Your planets, Your moons, Your stars, You care about my house, my dirty carpets, my Bills' absence, my Ron's tears, my own confusions. You care . . . and You will deliver me from all those concerns . . . if I ask.*

I shook my head at the awesomeness of such a fact.

He was God of the universe—and I was afraid to trust Him with my streaked windows and empty boxes? How dumb can one human be! I looked up at the Almighty ruefully and grinned. We both knew the answer: Dumb as *me!*

And so I took my emotions in hand. I relaxed in God's promise to deliver me from "noisome pestilence." And instead of moping in worry, I played the "Hallelujah Chorus" fortissimo and Ron was blasted out of his lonely room to listen to it with me. Later we drank Cokes together and talked.

We were warm, loving, secure in God's promise of *deliverance.*

And, of course, there must be this epilogue although if you know anything of God, you know its contents already:

In God's way

In God's time (which has *never* once been mine!)

The house sold.

My brother, an expert packer, came to help fill boxes.

A lady was found who "did" windows, carpets, and under the refrigerator.

The play was successfully performed and the two Bills came home.

Ron's faith kept him smiling.

And the house in Denver received all our furniture with the grace of having been custom-made for those pieces.

"Surely He shall deliver thee from the snare of the fowler and from the noisome pestilence." Not protection *from* those unpleasant experiences, but redemptive *deliverance* as He stands within unpleasant experiences.

11

Goodbye, Yesterday!

We arrived in Denver.

I stood in the doorway that first night, throbbing with weariness.

Billy came and put his arms around me.

"Moddy better go to bed," he said.

As a child, I took "expression" classes. For a recital, I gave a reading entitled "Molly Whimper." My brother adopted the name for me. My children found it delightful and began using it. Ultimately it transformed into "Moddy" and that is the name they still use.

I leaned against my strong son and sighed.

"Oh, Billy, there is so *much* to do! Just look! The house is *filled* with boxes! The whole place is *covered* with boxes!'"

He tipped my chin in that tender way he has when he knows I'm extra-tired. "But there's more than just boxes, Moddy. There's a lot of love in there!"

My eyes filled with tears at his wisdom.

Of course!

In this alien, box-filled house, there was *already* "a lot of love in there!" My heart surged on an upbeat: *How good is God!*

Later when I wrote the above account in my journal, I penned these words:

Perhaps that incident leads me into Psalm 91:4 because it occurs to me that the meaning of "He shall cover thee with his feathers" could be here. I, of course, had assumed it was an image of protection guaranteeing untarnished bliss. Perhaps it really means that when one is ill, tired, facing impossible tasks, "He shall cover thee with his feathers" of incredibly beautiful blessings. Even then.

I was achingly tired that night but God, through my son, "covered me with his feathers" by spotlighting that this house, while box-filled at the moment, was already irradiated with vibrant, vital, throbbing, thrilling family love.

I look back and see, through all the life-shattering, that I was constantly "covered" with "his feathers" of blessing.

Bill moved from academia to a job where his lifelong dreams of using academic expertise in the dynamic arena of the church are reality.

Billy transformed his life-plans from law to the ministry.

Ron learned the most important lessons of his life and *used* the pain for spiritual growth.

We four shared heart-talks on levels never touched before.

We articulated emotions left unstated before.

And there is the constant joy of memory building!

When the children were little, we often played a game: Tell Me a Memory! Ron would giggle about the fun of sneaking up on his absorbed-in-TV brother and, in emulation of "The Three Stooges" (a program which I had to ban because of this very problem), Ron would clobber then unsuspecting Billy on the head with a frying pan!

Billy would recount his embarrassment when, on a visit to a new church family, an older son began cursing. His mother corrected him by saying: "Those are the preacher's sons."

And articulate Ron replied: "Oh, don't worry about it! Our dad told us there would be people like you!"

I wrote:

But "covered with feathers," we are still memory-building.

On the way to Denver, we went by a lake for one day. It was glorious in the moonlight. We giggled, shared anecdotes, and sang. I noted the four sets of footprints, side-by-side, in the sand. I knew the waves would come and cover where we walked. They would be lost. But the imprint of that moment of laughing, loving togetherness was our priceless memory forever.

What I'm trying to say is that there is so much God-joy here! So much glowing, magical, multi-colored splendor that is routinely overlooked, taken for granted. But when I pause to look for "His feathers," I find my life splashed in dazzling pools of His blessings, far too numerous to count.

The Scripture says "Jesus wept."
That means He understands
The tight pressure
Of the heavy heart;
The distorted way
The world looks
Through tears . . . Although there is no record
                     I believe that "Jesus laughed."
                     That means He understands
                     The need for joyful spirits
                     Singing in unrestrained abandon;
                     The radiant way
                     The world looks
                     Through smiles . . .
He shall cover thee with his feathers
Is a promise to comfort, surely;
But is it not also a promise
That, no matter the turn of circumstance,
There will always be a "covering"
Of joyous blessing
From His loving heart?
We have only to look and find.
There is a storm of unanswered questions in my life.
I find no profundity for the "whys."
I find no wisdom for the "hows."
I find no clues for the "whens."
But "covered with His feathers," I find joyous blessings abound.
Lord God, when I look at my life and see it deluged with packed boxes, may I have the good sense to look more closely and see that the

crowded place of impossible work is also CRAMMED with LOVE! Even though storm rages outside, help me to cuddle inside in the specific knowledge that You are "covering me with Your feathers" and each shimmering strand is a joyful love-gift in my life!

There are so many: Ron's music, Billy's expressiveness, Bill's laughter, the pink bedspread Eunice bought, the shelves of books I love, the family pictures, the satin flowers Carole made, the purple mountains outside my windows hulking their shoulders into the glowing quilt of many-colored sunset . . . "He shall cover thee with His feathers . . ."

Rage, stomp, growl, you storms of life. There is an internal "covering" of joyous blessing in my life that nothing external can touch. It is mine. It can change my whole mental outlook if I choose to look at each feather and understand its loving, gentle, God-given covering of me.

Frustrated by life? Often.

Beaten by life? Never.

No matter how bitter circumstances may become, He will cover me with His feathers and under His wings I shall trust.

When all was in place in the new house, Billy went to college. Ron went to high school. Bill went to work. I stayed at home.

That first morning, I sat at my window and wrote:

Goodbye, Yesterday.
I held you.
I loved you.
But now there is a New World
Which I, too, shall hold . . .
Which I, too, shall love . . .

My eyes misted as I thought of "yesterday." It had been such fun teaching collegians, directing plays, public speaking, doing scholarly research, counseling young minds, assisting the birth of writers, reading strained iambic pentameter, critiquing a senior's effort at playwriting, participating in youthful growth, opening new doors, new horizons, new challenges . . .

Yesterday had been exploding, jumping, leaping, frolicking, rocking, swinging, singing, winging, activity . . . and it was gone. Forever.

A tear trickled down each cheek in overflow. Gently I wiped them away.

"Under his wings I can trust," I whispered. "I know it is going to be all right."

I looked about the room. This small study replaced the multicolored beauty, the rushing whirl of vibrant music of the old carousel. There was a moment of regret. I knew that whatever God and I could carve out in this "new world," it would never mean to me what the active collegiate world had meant . . . and then a question came before me: *Was it ever intended to?*

Surprised, I considered the question as another emotion surged in, ushering out the regret. The emotion grew to such dimension that I could feel nothing else: An awareness, an assurance that while something was over forever, something else had just begun.

Suddenly I understood that if the new seemed unequal to the old, it might be because . . . *the two were not to be compared!*

Circumstance had upheavelled my life-plans. But those circumstances were *redeemable.* How? I had not the faintest notion.

I could see how God had creatively used the dead carousel for the good of Bill . . . for the good of Billy . . . for the good of Ron . . . but me? Me? That still remained a mystery.

Yet I was "under his wings" and there I knew that although I could not *understand,* I could *trust!*

And in that moment, I felt a great excitement . . . for, in a flash of insight, it seemed to me that something might be ahead which grew out of the past, yes . . . but was totally different! This "something" might be deeper, fuller, more meaningful than anything in the past! This "redemption" of my life-plans might enable me to find my way, in an unparalleled manner, to the richness, the mercy, the immeasurable love of God.

"Under his wings" I would trust.

"Goodbye, Yesterday," I whispered. "I held you. I loved you."

My voice took on a surge of strength. I could feel reverberations of "The Hallelujah Chorus" in my tones as I said aloud:

"But now . . . there is a New World which I, too, shall hold
. . . which I, too, shall love . . ."

O You Redeemer God! my soul exulted. *Your Presence with me in all of life is enough. I have no need for promises of undisturbed bliss. I have something infinitely more precious in Your promise of redemption of unpleasant, even tragic, circumstance, Your promise of rebuilding a broken life, Your promise of a new world to replace the old. Thank You, Redeemer God.*

12

My God, My God!
Why Hast Thou
Forsaken Me?

The days began to turn in the new world.

To Ron, in his huge, alien high school in the strange big city, I wrote this poem:

> *If I could*
> *I would croon reality away*
> *With cradlesongs . . .*
> *We would gently rock*
> *And weep bewilderment*
> *Together . . .*
> *But . . .*
> *You are beyond my reach.*
> *His truth must be*
> *Your shield and buckler . . .*
> *It's just you*
> *And the "most High"*
> *Together now.*
> *No mommies allowed.*

I wept when I wrote it.

Not only for Ron, but for me.

I was caught in an illness that I had to learn to live with. It was all up to me. I was beyond the reach of doctors, family, or friends. It was just me and the "most High"—together now. *No mommies allowed* . . . even for me.

That essential human loneliness in facing responsibility is difficult in all ages, in all stages. But Ron and I both determined to try. Each in our own way. Each in our own arena.

Ron did well.

And then . . . there was me . . .

At the time of the first crisis when I had so resoundingly proven my lack of understanding of "limitations," my beloved career and my secure locale were taken from me. Although I complied with all of that, my doctors still predicted early death.

"I will try," I said earnestly.

"You will try very hard," replied the doctor who had come to know me well. "But you will fail. You speak articulately and with knowledge from your head. Your heart does not believe, for a moment, that it really applies to you."

He was right.

We moved to Denver.

I tried "very hard."

I failed.

The iron will power that had controlled all of my life went into gear in this exciting new world. From long habit, my mind began to spin with ways that my expertise could be used in this church, and my enthusiasm ran rampant. I began racing ever-faster and, as before, when my body issued warnings, I only lectured myself sternly, geared up my determined will power, and, as prophesied, hurled myself directly back into crisis.

Twelve weeks after our move to the *new world,* I lay in ICU with machines on all sides of me, monitoring the "vital" elements and understood, truly understood, that this was all *for real.*

My doctor stood beside me, tears in his eyes, and explained the damage to the body, the close proximity of death, and I could find no words to say. I could find no thoughts to think. It was as if an electric bolt had entered my skull and mesmerized me. All the funny medical jargon somehow had to be defined on levels *other* than the mind.

I had tried.

Only God knew how hard I had tried.

But it hadn't worked.

A lifetime of hyperactivity, overachievement, ironclad will power left me totally baffled in the face of my choices.

"Find another way to live, Ruth, or you will die."

My mind simply wouldn't move.

There was no referent that I could apply.

I truly did not *know* what these medical men were talking about. I only knew one way to define life: riotous activity. Any other interpretation so boggled my understanding that I was frozen in mental immobility.

I listened to my doctor explaining, explaining, explaining . . . and the only image he offered me of life was that of a "little old lady" tottering about her house caring for ivy! The idea was abhorrent in every dimension. I was a young, professional Ph.D. with responsibilities to care for my family and give service to others with my expertise. All this talk of a "little old lady" left me irritated and confused.

But the gravity in my doctor's eyes, the sounds of the machines in the room, the memory of the ripping pain made me know that irritation and confusion held no answer.

"I can't live like that any more," the nurses said I whispered in that first crisis. And I hadn't tried.

I truly had limited my parameters in those twelve weeks in Denver. There was impressive contrast when you placed life at the college in juxtaposition with my activity level in the new arena.

I had made changes.

But not enough.

I had tried. Very hard.

But I had failed.

Life "like that" was impossible. I had now proven that life "like this" was beyond my reach.

I lay very still as the great grief stormed my heart. I had struggled and suffered before as my career and hometown were blasted from me. I had tasted grief, but this time I could not delude myself. This grief was endless: a taste, bitter as aloes, that would never leave my mouth.

Life or death? Life as I understood it and early death. Somehow I must find life-changing wisdom that would affect every definition, perception, activity I held dear . . . and live longer in "limited parameters." My entire hierarchy of values would have to be restructured. The total essence of self-image would have to be reexamined and changed.

My doctor had told me it was probably impossible. I had proved him right. If I survived this crisis, would I take that "impossible task" as my quest?

Sorrow shook me with both hands; my mind burrowed like a squirrel with a nut. It was all unacceptable. I had tried to understand and make changes before. As it was now presented, I had only touched the surface.

Whirling giddily through life collecting gold trophies, silver plaques, degrees, and awards, I had thought those things my only *value*. Who, now *who*, would find any worth in the "little old lady"?

It was all so absurd!

So excruciatingly, agonizingly, torturously absurd!

I remembered a poem one of my contemporaries in graduate school had written:

> All is absurd, so let us laugh.
> Everything is phony, so let us
> Clink the glasses
> And laugh:
> The crazier, the better;
> The more ribald, the more rewarding!
> Life is an abyss of perdition;
> At its bottom is the reality
> Of despair;
> And while we sink into its tentacles,
> Let us laugh
> And refine the gall with cleverness,
> Lighten the darkness with brilliant
> Witticisms:
> Shallow they may be
> But at least
> We go down
> Laughing!

Such bravado had been unattractive to me in those years. It repelled me now.

No. I would not, could not accept the hollow answer of absurdity for life's mystery. True, every angle of the picture of my life seemed *absurd,* but there simply had to be more!

"He that dwelleth in the secret place of the most High . . ."

I drew a deep breath.

In my journal work, I had come to understand that phrase to mean the Redeemer God would be with me, in all of life, even absurdity such as this. He would not waste; He would find creative *use.*

So. I would pray.

I tried.

But all that came was a clutter of agitated words, phrases, petitions . . . all of them begging *a change of verdict from God!*

For the sake of Bill!

For the sake of Billy!

For the sake of Ronnie!

O *God!* my heart shrieked . . . *For the sake of Ruth!*

And there was no answer.

I looked about the room.

I wanted some dramatic miracle. I wanted the machines to begin registering some amazing body-change. I wanted a Damascus Road experience where confusion was changed to clarity.

Nothing happened.

The machines whirred.

The weakness enveloped.

Nothing happened. At all.

And then I understood. I was not only humanly alone in this agony of life-gone-totally-crazy. I was totally alone! And from the utter devastation of my soul, I cried:

"My God, my God, why hast thou forsaken me?"

The words echoed and re-echoed in the empty room. There was no answer. Depression descended and enshrouded me in a cubicle from which I could not reach out.

The nurse came and gave me a shot.

I lay quietly but every beat of my heart was screaming: *My God, my God, why hast thou forsaken me?*

Finally sleep overcame. As I slept, there was a dream. It was of the God-Man hanging on a wooden cross calling out in stark human anguish: "My God, my God, why hast thou forsaken me?"

When I awoke, the dream remained real. And my stunned mind began to move . . . slowly, fumblingly, but with *activity*.

This circumstance (*whatever* it was . . . for its dimensions and definitions, after *all* the medical lectures, were still unclear to me) . . . this imprisoning iron bond on my life was my reality. I had prayed for freedom. It had not come. I had prayed for a shining, glorious miracle to bind the brokenness and make me whole. Nothing happened.

And now I felt the most naked alienation of my life. In that small ICU room, *I was alone!*

But the dream had reminded me that there was One who had been in this same place in *human* experience. There was One who had, Himself, been broken, bent, thrust into the total despair of aloneness and forsakenness.

In my dream, I had relived the biblical record of the God-Man who had shouted my own cry from the shuddering depths of His soul: *My God, My God, why hast thou forsaken me?*

So I could never be alone.

There was One who understood *what it was like* to be caught in human existence with all its absurdity, its terror, its hopelessness. He had tasted the bitterness of this moment for Himself.

And He stood in this small room with me as the universal cry of alienation ripped from my whole being: *My God, my God . . . why?*

He understood. He had uttered that cry from the pain-quivering chasm of His soul. He had experienced the emotions of despondency, abandonment, betrayal, alienation, *fear*.

Later, as I recorded this moment, I wrote to the God/Man this letter:

I'm sorry You had to endure the agony of earthly sorrows. I'm sorry You had to discover the distorted way life looks through burning tears. I'm sorry You had to be wounded . . . but thank You . . . thank You for sharing it with me.

Thank You, Lord Jesus, for coming to earth
Thank You, Lord Jesus, for Your human birth;
Thank You for sharing my knowledge of tears
Thank You for sharing the terror of fears.
Thank You for sharing pain's dark rendezvous.
Thank You for sharing dreams that don't come true
Thank You for sharing loneliness stark
Thank You for sharing a world all gone dark.
Thank You for sharing this heart-ripping plea:
My God, my God, why hast thou forsaken me?
Why hast thou
Why hast thou forsaken
Forsaken . . . me?
Thank You, Lord Jesus, for sharing that cry with me.
Thank You, Lord Jesus, for sharing that pain with me.

In that small ICU room, there had been no thunder or lightning. There had been no astonishing miracle. There had been *nothing* to please my drama-loving heart.

And there had been no words.

Oh, how I *craved* words. Words clarified. Words justified. Words explained.

But there were none.

Only the sound of medical machines to break the silence. No words.

But the God/Man was there. He experientially understood.

A sudden light splashed my mind.

I had demanded words since the first moments of my life-carousel-burning. *God! Explain Yourself!*

And when there had been no words, I had taunted: *Why are You silent, Creator God? Would You rather not admit to the mess You have made? And if You deny creating the agonies coming from natural law and free choice, why do You consent to all that happens . . . and how? God! Explain Yourself!*

But He remained unspeaking. I could have been talking to a stone about my grief.

Now it occurred to me that words were redundant.

God had not created a world in which natural law and man's

free choice were operant, and then gone into eclipse. He had entered into the human scene in a human life. A woman contorted with pain giving birth to a Child who houses divine omnipresence and omnipotence in earthly form.

Angels sang: "Glory to God in the highest" in the miracle of God's becoming man. Simultaneous was a loud lamentation and mourning as Herod Antipas ordered all Jewish males under the age of two years slain. Thus, even in birth, there was the presence of grief of man as man.

God was born nude and vulnerable into the world where death, despair, injustice, insecurity are woven into the very fabric of life. He became indigenous to earth experiences of cruelty, betrayal, pain.

My demand for words was superficial. God did not need to *explain* human existence. He entered into human existence and lived it broadly. He compressed His eternal Self to the time space of one human life experiencing all life's joy, all life's sorrow, all life's beauty, all life's terror. God as man had been *utterly broken* on a cross and traversed the total despair of alienation and abandonment.

As I had cried: My God, my God, why hast thou forsaken me?, so had He. And that fact annihilated my needs for words of explanation. God had experienced human suffering. He understood and was *with* His creation *in* its pain.

I could not pass lightly over that God-Man cry of desolation: My God, my God, why hast thou forsaken me? because it was that cry that now illuminated my personal darkness. Yes. It did.

That cry smashed my superiority to the One whose omnipotence would prevent His understanding helplessness. That cry shattered my simpering arrogance that God could not possibly comprehend torturous pain. That cry slivered my demands for words, for He was given no words.

To bridge the abyss between time and eternity, the God-Man went *into* the abyss. He knows what it's like there. And that fact silenced my defiance and despair. And . . . that fact called me to redemption.

Redemption of sin. Redemption of circumstance.

I remembered that Malcolm Muggeridge had written that

"Christianity, from Golgatha onwards, has been the sanctification of failure." I had not had a glimmer of what he meant by that assertion.

Because its meaning eluded me, it tossed about in my brain from time to time. But there never was illumination.

Now it came to me with a shaft of light.

In a way, the God-Man on that cross was an affront to human values. The gods created by the Greeks and all other men are Herculean colossal heroes. Stunningly triumphant over all obstacles. Glorious. Supermen.

This penniless, helpless, suffering God-Man on Golgotha's cross was an antithesis to the great hero. Instead of stunning triumph, He testified in His human nature to human suffering and in His divine nature asserted that the Father God loved His creation *in* its suffering.

So . . . perhaps Muggeridge had been stating that in Jesus' earthly failure lay the seeds of reality, hope, *redemption*. Yes. Redemption. Rebirth.

What does one do when one experiences great grief?

Surely the best answer does not come in *words*. It comes in the God-Man who journeyed human tragedy before us.

The long road of sorrow, insight, healing, redemption, rebirth for any human person has already been trod in the sorrow, insight, healing, redemption, rebirth of Jesus Christ. We may walk *in His steps*.

God became flesh and blood and lived as a man. His flesh was torn. His blood was shed. For man. And at that moment, God conversed with man *in* His Son on the cross. God's complete answer.

13

Utterly Broken

Laurens Van der Post wrote: "One of the most pathetic things about us human beings is our touching belief that there are times when the truth is not good enough for us; that it can and must be improved upon. We have to be utterly broken before we can realize that it is impossible to better the truth. It is the truth that we deny which so tenderly and forgivingly picks up the fragments and puts them together again."

Utterly broken.

That is where I found myself.

I had refused the truth of my illness in every way my imaginative mind could devise. Intellectually, I had worked with it. But deep inside, I was sure it was "not good enough." With marvelous creative details, I gave the Lord graphic blueprints of how "the truth" could be—*must be* improved upon.

Now I was *utterly broken.*

Perhaps it was time for me to at least consider the possibility that I could not "better the truth." Every corpuscle resisted. Every thought-wave shuddered. Every emotion crouched and hid in spasms of pain.

My doctor is an extraordinary physician. He spent hours in discussion with Bill, with my sons, and with me.

But he understood that there had been many medical lectures from other doctors. None had ever touched me. Inside. I simply could not believe, accept this illness *as mine*. I had lived a lifetime by will power. Not to do so now seemed to me to be a cop-out.

Always the epitome of patience, he had listened, debated, asserted, cajoled, pleaded. One afternoon, he reached an explosion point and said curtly: "The choice is yours, Ruth. Make up your mind. Either be a 'cop-out' or a *corpse!*"

He turned on his heel and left the room.

Before my tears could wake in the shock of his anger, he was back. His face filled with compassion, his voice threaded with gentleness: "Please face the truth, Ruth. Please find a way to *live!*"

He picked up an envelope lying on my table. He wrote on it and handed it to me.

"Read that over and over until it is imprinted on your mind. This *is* your crossroads."

I took the envelope and he went away.

In red ink, he had written: "This illness is a documented fact in your life: one which cannot be changed. It is with you for life—or death—whichever you choose."

We have to be utterly broken before we can realize that it is impossible to better the truth. It is the truth that we deny which so tenderly and forgivingly picks up the fragments and puts them together again.

Could my "truth" do that for me?

I had no idea how. I had no idea why.

Later my slender, hurting, blond teen-ager Ron slipped into the room. He ruffled my hair. His hands caressed my face.

"The doctor asked me what I would do if you died," he whispered to me. "I told him I'd kill myself."

Tears jerked in my eyes as I grabbed his hand.

"Ron! No!"

He snuggled his wet face into my shoulder as he cried: "Oh, Moddy, if you're not in my world, I don't want to live!"

The nurse brought in a telephone.

From the campus in another state, my college-senior Billy sobbed in heartbreak. Friends had written that they had tried to "reach out" to him at this time. "But he walks so strong," they said. "How can you reach out to someone who *always* smiles?"

As I listened to his agony spurting out in tearful words over the telephone lines, I knew this brave young man needed a mother in his life. Outwardly competent, he inwardly drew strength from the earthly presence of his mother.

Bill came in. Like Billy, he was "walking strong" as always. Like Billy, he was smiling.

He handed me a card.

It read:

> *It's a lonely world*
> *When I'm not with you.*

Under the printing, he had scribbled:

> *This card says it:*
> *I need you!*
> *Bill*

I looked at this professional, controlled, invulnerable Ph.D. and knew he needed a wife as much as had the skinny, non-professional, vulnerable kid I had married.

We have to be utterly broken before we can realize that it is impossible to better the truth. It is the truth that we deny which so tenderly and forgivingly picks up the fragments and puts them together again.

Could my "truth" do that for me?

I had no idea how. I now had a crystal-clear idea *why.*

Three men needed me in their world.

That was enough.

I picked up the small envelope. "Life—or death," it challenged. "Whichever you choose."

Aloud, I said: "Whichever you choose. I choose life. With the illness . . . I choose life. In limited parameters . . . I choose life. Whatever . . . *whatever* that might possibly mean!"

I buried my face in my hands.

My mind circled like an animal in a trap.

What is life "with the illness?" What *is* life "in limited parameters?" *What is life?*

The question rocked like a treadmill to which I was bound. What could a human creature know of life? A human creature whirling, pirouetting, rushing with activity until grief ripped apart the veil and I saw my naked, shivering self within, staring out at life like a river running swiftly downhill.

I had "chosen" life before.

I had said all the right things before.

Somehow I understood that I had to make inner shifts, mental adjustments on levels untouched before.

I was willing . . . I *was* willing . . . but I had not the faintest idea *how* to begin.

One afternoon, I had strained for comprehension.

My doctor and Bill had been discussing monitors of strength, boundary-holders to my enthusiasms. It all congealed into the dreadful "little old lady" that was the most abhorrent image I had ever beheld.

They were discussing the possibilities that I might continue with my writing. Their voices swirled about me until it finally dawned on me that they actually were *solemnly* suggesting that I might write with an *alarm clock on my desk!* When it rang, at the end of an hour or two (whatever limit was chosen), then I would totter off to bed like a good "little old lady" should!

I looked at these two grown men seriously considering such idiocy. Didn't they know that in the rush of creativity I could write all day, all night? Bill had been with me in a time when, in a vast outpouring of enthusiasm (and need to meet a deadline), I had written an entire book without sleeping. Bill had brought my meals to the desk. He had understood my lack of fatigue, my total containment in the creative act. He had never chided me. He had paced it with me.

And now he sat, without laughter, as a doctor actually talked of ringing an alarm clock to send me to bed after an *hour* of typing? The creative juices would only then be beginning. No writer would walk away because an *alarm clock sounded!*

My shrill laughter stopped their conversation.

When I explained to them the ridiculous dimension of their concept, Dr. Madden reached for the envelope and handed it to me. Very quietly he asked: "Do you want to live?"

My eyes filled with tears of frustration. I was caught in a vise of terror.

Didn't they understand? They were sitting there in quiet conversation . . . *calmly destroying me!*

Pain clutched freshly at my heart and, with all the scathing sarcasm I could muster, I charged: "I suppose you really want me to spend the rest of my life in a rocking chair!"

"No, Ruth," he said, his voice an odd combination of wistfulness and resignation. "I am convinced that unless you find *life-changing* wisdom deep inside *you* . . . that even if I tied you in a rocking chair forcing you to be the 'little old lady' you dread so much, you would rock yourself to death. *You* have to learn about stillness. *You* have to discover serenity. Inside."

Both men were so kind that I tried to wall up my grief in a secret part of my heart until they would go away. It was so sore there, so pulpy to the touch, that I dared not expose it even to these gentle eyes.

And so I waited.

They finally went away together.

When the door closed, the stress of it all became unbearable and I released the floodgate of my tears. I lay on my back, pounded the bed, and almost drowned in the Niagara of sobs that shook my tormented frame.

"Life-changing wisdom . . . deep inside of you."

Yes. Yes.

But *how* did one find it? *How?*

When finally I could cry no more, I knew I had come to the end. I had to find assistance.

Totally helpless, irrevocably beyond human aid, I did something I had never done before. Or since.

I looked at the heavy door to my room.

And I prayed: *Doctors have walked through that door. Bill has walked through that door. All have tried to help. But they cannot. I need 'life-changing wisdom' and it cannot come from a human source. Lord God, I am dependent on you.*

Because my need is great, I am asking that You walk in that door. I am asking that You give me some gesture, some sign, some assurance that You really are working with me and that, in Your time, in Your way, 'life-changing wisdom' will come to me.

O Redeemer God, come to me. Please come to me.

My eyes were on the door.

Immediately it opened.

Barbara, the nurse who had been in charge since my admittance, walked in. In one hand, she carried a rose. In the other, she carried a much-worn book.

She came to the bed and placed the rose on the table. She still held the book.

"Ruth," she said quietly, "I want to tell you something that I think is important."

I looked at her curiously as I tried to wipe away the traces of my tears.

"A lady just came to the desk and asked for me. She introduced herself and explained that although she had never met you, she felt close to you. When she heard you were here, she wanted to reach out to you. She knew she could not come in, so she brought a rose as a token of her esteem and gratitude to you. And she brought this book so you could see for yourself why you are important in her life."

I frowned in bewilderment.

"You wrote a book about your faith in God?" she asked.

I nodded.

"This lady read it. It has been so meaningful in her life that she has written throughout this book its messages to her. She said she wanted you to see the parts that had made *the* difference in her life."

Barbara handed me the book.

Tears streamed down her cheeks. "Oh, Ruth," she said in her love-husky voice, "doesn't this give you *hope?* Here is a lady who read a book you wrote years ago and her life was changed for the better. The impact of your life goes on even while you lie here in a hospital bed. Even to people you have never seen."

Barbara took my hand. She had been with me in my struggle and she understood my hopelessness.

Now she urged: "Ruth, doesn't this give you *hope?*"

Tears were stumbling down my crusty cheeks as I held the book. I whispered, "Yes, Barbara. It gives me hope. But it gives me more. You see, this lady didn't come to the hospital at *this* moment accidentally. You didn't come with her message just as a happenstance. Barbara, in the instant of my direst extremity, when I *had* to have help . . . through the lady . . . through you . . . God came to me."

When she left the room, I looked at the worn book in awe. Slowly I opened it.

This is what I read:

> Grateful am I for the times when in response to my request for light, He gave me the dark. For it was there, helpless, frightened, completely dependent, I realized my own inadequacies and my deep need of God. I understood better that, without Him, I was nothing. I wanted to know and see, but He knew that in the dark I would learn lessons which would escape me in the busyness and fulfillment of light.

And I cried.

Not in desperate frustration. But in the knowledge that the "most High," the Redeemer God had, indeed, come through that heavy door and given me a tangible sign of His Presence *with.* He had known my last erg of strength had evaporated. I *had* to hear from Him. And He reached out to me in a tangible way.

I had been felled.

I would never teach again; never direct another play; never speak at another convention; never present another paper at an academic workshop . . . I might never write another book . . . but I had invested those years of activity. Although I lay still, my students were utilizing the skills I had shared . . . and the books and plays I had written were still being used by God, even now in the life of this lady whose name I didn't know.

That was comforting. But it was a "grace note" to God's answer to my heart-cry.

That was all impressive and I was deeply grateful . . . but . . . it provided *no life-changing wisdom* by which to live.

What I had done in other days was gone from me. The problem confronting me now was a future that was totally incomprehensible. Stare into it with all the intensity I could muster, I could find nothing but *dark.*

My eyes returned to the passage underlined in the lady's worn book. I had written those words twelve years before.

I had known darkness, yes . . . but *never* any darkness like *this!*

I studied the words. I had written them at age twenty-nine.

My heart felt a pang of bitterness. What did I know of darkness at twenty-nine?

I must have dashed these off glibly . . . and then I stopped . . . remembering that young woman. I remembered the study where she typed; the circumstances of her life.

No. They were not glib.

Darkness at twenty, twenty-five, twenty-nine had been terrifying . . . for it was my first exposures. I could not, then, have borne the intensity of the darkness I was experiencing now. So although young and relatively inexperienced in suffering, I had written Truth. The "most High" had "stepped aside" to allow experiences of ever-deepening darkness through the years . . . so I would not be whammed by events beyond my capacity to bear.

Now, twelve years later, with life splattered all about me, I asked for "life-changing wisdom" . . . and He gave it to me. In my own words.

Oh, it was *not* the "life-changing wisdom" I wanted!

Not for a moment!

I had mentally offered up beautifully-detailed ways that God could right my world. All of them were stunningly dramatic and, in one fell swoop, washed away all pain and erased darkness with glorious sunshine.

Were He to follow my gladly-given instructions, His life-changing wisdom would have made the blackness golden in the twitch of a nose! That was *my* definition of life-changing wisdom.

As usual, He ignored my helpfulness and went on with His divine redemptive work. And when I had to have *words* from Him to hold me steady, they were:

Grateful am I for the times when in response to my request for light He gave me the dark. For it was there helpless, frightened, completely dependent, I realized my own inadequacies and my deep need of God . . . I would learn lessons which would escape me in the busyness and fulfillment of light.

I took a deep breath.

I understood.

There were going to be *no* abracadabra miracles!

There was going to be *no* stunning drama!

There was going to be *nothing* instantaneous. I was still in the dark. And I would have to walk in that blackness with Him, helpless, dependent, aware of my need of Him . . . knowing that, in that unpleasant groping journey, I would "learn lessons which would escape me in the busyness and fulfillment of light."

He would not deliver me *from* the brokenness of my world. He would *use* the brokenness in His way, in His time.

14

To Reach
for God

I do not understand about divine healing.

It is a phenomenon that remains an insoluble mystery to my mind.

As word of my illness spread through my nationwide community of friends, I was deluged with books, letters, tapes—all demanding my instant healing. One minister called long-distance to tell me that I was *guaranteed* roaring good health on a wooden cross 2,000 years ago. It was my *right* as a Christian.

I read. I listened. I prayed.

Some well-meaning people wrote detailed letters, outlining the contributions I was prepared to make to society, and then inferring, if not specifically asserting, that I was a cop-out if I did not "become well" and use my expertise as it was needed.

Others reprimanded me for my lack of faith which would surely make me instantly whole.

Some queried me in regard to sins for which I was being punished.

A lady, whose spiritual stature I admired inordinately, shared with me her experience. She had an incurable, debilitating illness. One night, she was praying and saw Jesus literally appear before her eyes. He reached out His hand, touched her, and immediately she was whole.

X-rays and lab reports confirmed it.

Returning strength underlined it.

Her vibrant life of service left no doubt. She had been healed.

I rejoiced with her.

But I knew the rejoicing was not what she wanted from me. She was anticipating that I would have the same experience.

Wistfully I yearned for it.

Beseechingly I prayed for it.

Conscientiously I met every biblical condition I understood.

But it did not happen. And I could not lie.

Her disappointment in me drove my spirits into an abyss of depression. I had done everything I, humanly, could know to do. When my friend had done those things, an amazing miracle occurred. When I did those things, the darkness swirled about me. There was no vision of Jesus. No tangible touch of divinity. No surging of God-given strength.

Nothing.

A total stranger called one day.

She said: "I want to quote a Scripture to you from Psalm 91." My interest piqued immediately—"my" Scripture!

She repeated: "Because thou hast made the Lord, which is my refuge, even the most High, thy habitation; There shall no evil befall thee, neither shall any plague come nigh thy dwelling" (Ps. 91:9-10).

She asked if I knew the passage. I assured her that I did.

"Well, then," she said with authority, "why aren't you using it?"

"I don't understand," I told her.

"From what I read of your writings and hear of your character, you have made the Lord your habitation."

"I have tried with all my heart," I assured her.

"Well, then, you have the promise that no evil shall befall you; no plague shall come nigh. You have only to *claim* that to be well. If you remain ill, it is because *you want to!*"

I gasped with shock.

She went on without notice.

"Divine healing is just like conversion. You have to be willing to accept it before it can be yours. Obviously, to this point, you have been unwilling to receive what God wants for you."

I gulped. I felt like I had been kicked in the stomach. Or slapped very hard.

Realizing she had my full attention, she said: "Now I want you to bow your head instantly. Ask God to forgive you for not being healed before this. And demand that He keep His promise."

I was so stunned by the lady's words that I could not speak.

She became irritated. "What are you waiting for?" she snapped. "You know this promise is yours. Now demand that God take the evil out of your life. Now."

When I still did not respond, she almost shouted: "What is the matter with you? I am trying to help you!"

"I know that," I answered slowly. "I appreciate your interest and concern. It is just that I do not feel I have the right to *demand* anything from God."

"But He promised . . ." she began.

"He promised 'no evil, no plague' that is *irredeemable*. He promised 'no evil, no plague' that He cannot 'work together for good'. But what He allows to enter my life and how He chooses to redeem it has to be His choice . . . not mine."

Thoroughly disgusted with me, she made a few harsh remarks and hung up the phone. I lay for a long time considering the verse.

Could the lady be right? I asked myself.

Was I being denied because I did not demand?

Jesus Christ did not demand relief from suffering. He entered into human existence in its entirety. He hungered; was thirsty; was disappointed in friends who slept when He cried; was betrayed by one He trusted. He submitted to the agony of crucifixion. He died a painful human death. He did not *demand* what His human heart must have desired.

Earlier, in the sermon on the Mount, He had said: "Blessed are they that mourn, for they shall be comforted." He was attesting that many times in life we are called upon to *mourn*. He made no statement that we could *demand* immunity to sorrow which caused our hearts to mourn. Instead He promised that *when* we mourned we should be comforted.

No. Jesus Christ had set the pattern for life with God. Although I prayed for a miracle, I simply could not believe I had the right to demand my own way!

Confusion over my dilemma swelled and seethed in increasing dimension. Finally the senior pastor of our church dedicated an entire Sunday evening to the problem.

In his sermon, he stated that, at the conclusion, he would ask all to gather about the altar for prayer that my life be returned to me. Then he asserted that there were three ways God could answer that volume of prayer.

He could say no. And I would slip over into the Other World.

He could say yes. I would be immediately revitalized, with all damage to the body instantly corrected.

He could say: "No instant answer is My will. Wait and let Me work."

In my bed, alone, I prepared myself spiritually for that service with an earnest intensity. Only God had known the depths of human agony my soul had endured because of this illness. Only God understood how fully I yearned to race back into life with the service of my whole heart. Only God knew . . .

But the pressure from so many who did not share my interpretation of Scripture made me strive with painstaking detail to be sure I was as open to His will as I knew how to be.

When the hour of unified prayer for me approached, confusion still swirled within me. Nudges that I should be doing something different, something startling, something *demanding* plagued me. But . . . when I felt it was time for me to open my heart in prayer with those of my friends in the church . . . I found that the only prayer I could pray was one structured upon that of Jesus in Gethsemane. I felt I had no right to pray any other kind of prayer.

Scripture tells us His soul was in agony.

So was mine.

As He prayed then . . . so I prayed now.

Father, all things are possible to Thee . . .

Ah yes! I know about the marvelous healing of my friend to

whom Jesus appeared in a vision. I know my sister-in-law had an appalling plague of eczema on both hands which was instantly healed in a moment of prayer. Scripture abounds with record of physical miracles when natural law was countermanded.

I do know . . . I do believe . . .

"Father, all things are possible unto thee . . ."

"Remove this cup from me . . ."

O . . . my heart swelled until I thought it would surely burst from my body. O . . . Father . . . please, please, please *"remove this cup from me" . . .*

I took a deep breath and waited.

Nevertheless, not what I will, but what thou wilt. . . . Jesus had said next. . . . The most difficult words in the English language *. . . and* the most necessary.

How hideously painful to form those words! My lips halted; my tongue moved woodenly; even my teeth ached.

I summoned all my strength, understanding full well all that was implied. . . . And then I said . . . gasping, choking, hurting . . . I said: *Nevertheless, not what I will, but what thou wilt.*

And deep inside, where the meanings are, the Redeemer God said two words: "Trust Me."

Only three times in my life have I truly felt the most High give an articulated message in the "secret place" of my being. I have often had words impressed on my mind that I felt came directly from His heart. I have often received divine communiques in other ways.

But only three times has there been this special, direct, incontestable communication that I felt God was speaking *directly* to me.

The first time, He said: "I want Bill to go back to school and I will make a way."

And He did.

The second time, He said: "Your plans are not Mine." And to my utter astonishment, He proceeded to turn us from our planned path onto a new road of graduate school. And His plans were better than ours.

Now . . . after such a long silence in this ongoing illness, there came this gentle, tender, love-lined message: "Trust Me!"

And, in tears I told Him that I had/did/would.
And that was all.

The next week, I wrote to my friend, Pat Wellman, this account:

"I cannot explain it. I cannot understand it.

"As the doctor brooded yesterday over the test results, I lay on his table and thought about Sunday night. The storybook ending would have been a medical report of a reborn gland and all damage corrected. But my physician was somberly talking about the 'exquisite tragedy' of imminent death.

"I, the word-loving person, was impressed with the juxtaposition of those two words.

"I, the rational person, understood he was talking about *me*.

"I, the child of God, knew that the 'most High' who said to me Sunday night: 'Trust Me!' is a Redeemer of circumstance who can turn any 'tragedy' into triumph . . . if we allow.

"Oh, Pat, I am trying, with all my being, to 'allow.' I *do* want His will to be done.

"And so, this week, I lie very still. 'Trust Me!' He said. That I can and will do . . . and the long lonely hours move in a peaceful serenity that passes all understanding.

"I, the articulate, would like to explain it.

"I, the inquiring mind, would like to understand it.

"I, the exuberant spirit, would like to bound back into life.

"But, with all those now denied, I rest in the beautiful invitation He gave me Sunday night: 'Trust Me!' There I know that, whatever the future, I am secure."

15

Building a
New World

It was decided that the necessary "limited parameters" for me would be the walls of my home. My doctor erected a non-visible but sternly imposed "No Visitors" sign. One of my greatest enemies was talking. I had always communicated from top-of-hair to end-of-toenail. It took incredible strength. Such strength was no longer mine. "Visitors, even those who love you the most," my doctor said, "can kill you."

I, the gregarious, people-loving person who wanted to share my every thought in graphic detail with anyone who would listen, would build a *new world* inside those parameters. Now *there* would be a miracle!

I was so weak I could hardly walk from one room to another without assistance. I could rarely sit up for an entire meal. Reading was tiring. Often the noise of television was a strain.

It wasn't going to be easy, but I was determined. This new world would be my love-gift to my three men.

I had another determination. It could only be mine as a love-gift *from* the three for whom I was "living like this."

And so we had a conference.

I lay on the bed and the three men sat about me. We were very serious.

"I love you," I said and the tears came. I took a deep breath and forced them back. No strength allowed for tears. Every ounce of energy had to be spent on this plea. "I will attempt to prove my love for you by finding a way to be alive on this earth. Obviously my life will not touch any others, but *you three* are the vital ones. I will do my best to give you, Billy and Ronnie, a mother. I will do my best to give you, my darling Bill, a wife."

We were all choking on emotion. But I had to go on.

"Now. I want *you* to give a love-gift to me. That will be your promise that you will walk *free of me* in the world. *I* will be responsible for my limited world and whatever God and I shall make of it. *You* must promise that you will walk freely in *your* worlds to be all your hearts compel you to be."

I took Bill's face in my hands and kissed him. I tipped his chin to look gravely in his eyes: "What a tragedy it would be if your ministry for God to others would *in any way* be hampered because I did not want to be alone! As your love-gift to me, promise you will *never* feel me as a burden. Even when you feel concern for me . . . even when you feel a longing to be with me, even when you have a yearning to physically care for me . . . walk free. Walk free to be the minister God would have you to be. That would be your finest love-gift to me."

I took the hands of my sons. "You are growing, developing. There are many doors for you to enter, many adventures for you to understand, many challenges to explore. As *your* love-gift to me, walk free!"

I shushed their protests.

"God and I will create a new world for me . . . one in which I may be able to live for years. It won't be easy, but that is *my* challenge. And the doing of it is my love-gift to you."

I cocked my head in the way that always makes them smile, looked up through my lashes, and with my most wily female sorcery, asked: "Will you, sirs, give love-gifts to me?"

And we clung together on the bed . . . the four of us . . . weeping in promises and prayers for courage in facing the difficulties of giving these love-gifts to each other.

Anne Lindbergh expressed my feelings best:

> Him that I love I wish to be
> Free:

Free as the bare top twigs of tree,
Pushed up out of the fight
Of branches, struggling for the light,
Clear of the darkening pall,
Where shadows fall—
Open to the golden eye
Of sky;

Free as a gull
Alone upon a single shaft of air,
Invisible there,
Where
No man can touch,
No shout can reach,
Meet
No stare;

Free as a spear
Of grass,
Lost in the green
Anonymity
Of a thousand seen
Piercing, row on row;
The crust of earth,
With mirth,
Through to the blue,
Sharing the sun
Although,
Circled each one,
In his cool sphere
Of dew.

Him that I love, I wish to be
Free—
Even from me.

My three men gave the requested love-gift and went back
into their active, challenging, whirling worlds. I wore flannel
pajamas, lay "very still," and looked about me.

It was like a little nest, this room arranged so lovingly for my
every need while the men were gone. A little nest . . . and then
I remembered. . . . My husband, Bill, is unpoetic, prosaic,
down-to-earth, literal.

For the most part.

Occasionally, he surprises me.

When I was flown by ambulance plane to the diagnostic hospital in the first crisis, Bill sped across the ground in our car. When he arrived, they let him in ICU. He said that I lay, knees drawn up, huddling against the back far corner of my bed, as a bird huddles on a rocky ledge, too hurt to fly, yet starving. After a few moments, he said that he turned from the room, walked to the end of the hall, and leaned his head against the cold windowpane. He said there were a million lights blinking over the city below, but in each of them he could only see the tiny form of the wife he loved . . . whom illness now had caged from him . . . and he, who *never* displays emotion, cried.

The next day, he went downtown to a cafeteria to get away from hospital food. He passed a bookstore in the center of the mall. A book title caught his attention. It was *The Bird With the Broken Wing*. He went over and picked up the book and held it long in his hands. He said it seemed to describe what had happened to the girl he loved. She, the soaring, adventuring, free-wheeling bird, now lay with a broken wing. He said he put the book down and bypassing the cafeteria, hurried to the car, where he wept inconsolably. His "bird" had a broken wing. Even if I survived, one fact was ours. I would never fly again.

That image became vividly important to me. I lay in the small boundaries of my "nest" with a "broken wing" and wondered how one began "creating a new world."

I felt I had a strong foundation. My mind had done much good work in the last two years. Although I discovered that my spirit, my enthusiasms paid little heed to what my mind knew when I was in the thrilling arena of people, I had survived another crisis. I was being given another chance.

Bill had gotten me a new notebook. It was light blue, sprinkled with white puffs of clouds through which soared a regal eagle. I looked at it wistfully. I was "the bird with the broken wing." I would never fly again.

And then I remembered a passage I had memorized from Melville's *Moby Dick* long ago:

There is a wisdom that is woe; but there is a woe that is madness. And there is a Catskill eagle in some souls that can alike dive down into the blackest gorges, and soar out of them again and become invisible in the sunny spaces. And even if he forever flies within the gorge, that gorge is in the mountains; so that even in his lowest swoop the mountain eagle is still higher than other birds upon the plain, even though they soar.

My mind went back over the words: "There is a Catskill eagle in some souls that can dive down into the blackest gorges . . . (but) that gorge is in the mountains . . ."

"Bird with the broken wing" . . . limited to a nest in the "blackest gorges" of grief . . . but I *could choose* to dwell "in the mountains" so that there would still be the glories of height.

Depression stalked about in the lowlands. Defeat was quicksand in the bottoms. I would make my nest "in the mountains." I would strive to be "a Catskill eagle."

Isaiah may have had this exact image in mind when he wrote: "But they that wait upon the Lord shall renew their strength, they shall mount up with wings like eagles."

And so I opened the new notebook bearing the symbol of the soaring eagle and wrote my first lines:

It is God's way not to waste anything. I sit here in this lonely house in the dark, in the pain, in the finality of knowing that my 'old world' is gone with all its definitions, its value-hierarchies, and its expectations.

I resolve that, every day, I shall search for one way . . . and then another . . . and still one more way to allow God to make creative use of my tragedy. I refuse to be knocked down by this. I want to allow God to make redemptive use of my entire life.

There is a possibility, a very good one, that I shall not live through this year. I have no fear of death. I know it is only the door into the Larger Life. But so long as I can live on this earth with/for my three men, I shall do so with all the love of my heart.

And it is an opportunity to prove, as never before, what I have believed: that Jesus Christ Himself is Christianity. He got up and walked out of that tomb alive. He is here with me now. He is involved with me just as I am.

I prayed for a miracle. That did not happen. As God is realistic, so shall I be. I shall look at what is in this small room. And I shall find a way to create a new world.

I have no idea how. But Jesus Himself demonstrated on the cross that nothing ever needs to be wasted if He is on the scene. Calvary happened to Jesus, but He lived through it to create for us all the Resurrection, the Ascension, the coming of the Holy Spirit . . . a whole new dispensation, as the theologues call it . . .

From the darkness of Calvary, He surely can lead me through my darkness to a plateau where I can create a new world.

That was my first entry.

It was a good prologue. It set the tone. It pointed toward the goal. But it was not the beginning of an abracadabra! magical change.

I wrote those words. I adopted that stance. But my reality remained as limited, as black, as hopeless as ever. The psalmist succinctly summarized much of my journal entries when he wrote: "I am worn out with pain; every night my pillow is wet with tears."

As always, the psalmist was wise. I learned that giving vent to emotions is best. If you can yell and kick and beat the wall with your head, if you can pound with your fists and scream your grief, that is best. The more powerful the emotion, the stronger should be your venting of it. And if you allow yourself that release, it will enable you to recover more quickly. The emotion drains you to the point of exhaustion and, in that inert heap, you find that, deep inside, your spirit begins to pull itself together.

That may seem strange, but it is true. I can remember when the suffering would be so great that I would go in the closet, stuff a towel in my mouth so no one could hear me, and scream with all the intensity of my being. I responded like a wounded animal with no concern whatever for sophistication or civilization. Such total surrender to emotion released strains and tensions deep within. When it was over, there was an overwhelming relief, a yielding to some sort of inner acceptance of the destruction that had occurred.

I remember one time after such a storm of weeping, I pulled

myself over to look at the red-mottled-swollen face in the mirror
and I whispered in panic: O God, *what am I ever going to do?*
And from that inner strength that was forming inside, words
whispered back: "You'll build a new world where you will find joy
again."

I was incredulous. I stared at the image in the mirror in the
beginning of belief. It was a giant step into life on the *other* side
of broken dreams.

I would like to write out here a swift, easy formula for
building the "second half" of life when the first has been destroyed. Because I have found no such thing, I have none to
share.

I will try to glean from my journals some of the steps that led
from wound to healing. I will try to identify some of the specific
bricks that were used for the superstructure of my new world.

When my careers were taken from me, I felt like one of
those spiraled shells washed up on a beach. Poke a toothpick in
and around; you find nothing there. Whatever once lived inside
is now dead and gone.

I quickly discovered that our society is so structured that
most of us are valued for what we can *do*. And if there comes a
time when we can no longer do anything spectacular or meaningful, one not only loses a beloved world, one loses all self-
identity.

And so that is where I had to begin.

I had to try to discover who I was. Not Ruth—the one-
with-ten-talents. But simple-quiet-Ruth-inside.

It was hideously difficult.

I was hurtled into an identity crisis on top of my grief for a
personally lost world . . . a world that was able to move along
quite well without me, thank you! I was obviously *not* indispens-
able. Perhaps what I had contributed had been of little value
after all. Perhaps I had only been fooling myself to believe I had
significance in my careers.

Whether or not that were true, it no longer mattered. My
job no longer involved exploring the formal *vita* sheet, perusing a
trophy-laden cabinet, remembering external achievement.
Those were gone from me. Forever.

I had to release all that and turn inward. I had to see, touch, and come to understand the *who* of Ruth.

That was especially traumatic for me because my self-image was deeply rooted in the belief that my *value* was in the exterior vivacity, talent, competency. Stripped of all that, I had to find and accept the quiet essence of Ruth as valuable. The pain was like rending, tearing claws. Hideously ripping. Unending.

The knowledge that all that "was left" was a small plain person lunged at me, swiftly, blindingly, plunging through me like the beak of a hawk. It would have been impossible had God not been with me. But because I was certain He was there, there was hope and promise. He believed utterly in my worth to Him. I had fought that through and was now confident that His knowledge of "what was left" of Ruth was totally accurate. He knew the worst; He knew the best. In realistic proportion. He accepted me. So would I.

And so I took a deep breath and began to try to find self.

I had always been a *we*. I had always been connected intrinsically with another. I had been a daughter to beloved parents, wife to a racing idealistic young man, mother to two growing, challenging sons, minister's wife, public speaker, counselor, college professor.

Now it was time for me to be an *I*.

Even as an *invalid*. I believe *invalid* is a harsh and hurtful word. I did not want to be pigeonholed as an invalid. And yet I was. Even in magazine or newspaper headlines heralding one of my books or plays, I would be referred to in huge capital letters as INVALID. I understood that made good copy and people would read it, perhaps, more quickly than an article about an "ordinary" person. But it was still painful because it inferred invalidism as my chief value.

I wrote in my journal:

I am not a second-class citizen. I am not a nonentity. I am a wife; a mother; a concerned, vital, laughing, giving woman. I am a person, whole inside.

I am alive. I am part of the world. I have a handicap, surely. But don't most people? In some way?

No matter what other people call me, I shall not ever refer to myself as an invalid. I am not Ruth Vaughn, invalid. That is the body. That is not I. Inside, I am Ruth Vaughn, loving, needed mother of two; vibrant, needed wife to one glorious man. It would be nice to have all this in a strong body. But it is not essential. I have something better: I am me!

And in that journal entry, I laid the first brick of a new world. I accepted the fact that I was now an *I*. And *I* was important.

There is so much emphasis on humility and self-effacement that the Christian can often forget the admonition: "Love thy neighbor as thyself." As thyself. Not *better than*. Not *instead of*. *As thyself*. I had fallen into that trap. Now I had to work my way out of it and learn to love self.

And in that learning, I laid, perhaps, my second brick in a new world. I determined I would be my own best friend.

Does that sound strange? It is fact; we are often *our own worst enemies*. Because we make the wrong choices in answering questions we constantly face.

In my answers now, I understood that, as my own best friend, I would *choose* my impact on myself.

Would I lift self up when I fell low . . . or push her down?

Would I be a self-supporter . . . or her critic?

Would I do things, think thoughts, explore emotions to give self joy . . . or to make her cry?

I had not understood before the power I had in my own life.

I wrote in my journal:

1. I BELIEVE IN MY PERSONAL WORTH. Even now. When I am tempted to believe that my only function in life is to consume oxygen and use needed money from our family income, I will deny those thoughts. By an act of will, I refuse to think the unpleasant. By an act of will, I choose to daily believe I can always be a contributing member of my family, of my society. When I can sit up, I can reach out through my typewriter. When I have to lie down, my mind can still whirl and dart in creation. I can pray. Most of all, I can love.

2. *I WILL UNDERSTAND AND ACCEPT MY BODY. As
it is. I will care for it conscientiously. When it needs total rest, even
though my mind wants to do a million other things, I will give to the
body as needed. I will not strain against its limitations.*

3. WHEN I AM WEAK OR TIRED, I WILL NOT
THINK. *I have found that fearful, torturous thoughts can come in
mobs. Disorderly mobs. There are times when I have no business
trying to think. And so I determine that when strength and clarity are
not mine, I will not think.*

4. *I WILL REFUSE SELF-RECRIMINATION. Remorse is
a gaping pit into which it is easy to fall. But it is futile action. It is
beating oneself in a vain attempt to make what has happened unhap-
pen. (If only I had been wiser . . . if only I had tried harder . . . if
only I had listened more carefully . . . this might not have happened!)
Remorse is brutally unfair to self for it feeds on illusions just like living
on memories or holding mementos of the lost world continually. Remorse is dealing in illusions. I refuse it.*

5. *I WILL REFUSE ENVY. When I read or hear of my colleagues achieving wonderful pinnacles I have prepared myself to reach,
I refuse ever to say: "If only . . ." (If only this had not happened to
me, I would be going there, doing this, creating that. . . .) Like
remorse, it is futile action and changes nothing but my hurting feelings.
When the "feeling-sorry-for-me" syndrome hits, I will remember what
Jesus said to Peter when he questioned the Master about John: "What
is that to thee? Follow thou me." I know MY job is building a new
world. I have neither the strength nor time to deal in "what might have
been."*

6. *I WILL REFUSE THE WORD WHY? If it even flickers
on my brain's horizon, I will beat it with every club I can find. Only
when it is totally routed can acceptance come. And with acceptance
comes peace. I will never ask "Why?"*

7. *I WILL BE A COMPASSIONATE, CARING
ADULT-FRIEND TO MY TERRIFIED CHILD-SELF. Growing
up is not a one-way trip. The adult/child are not mutually exclusive. I
am both. It is all right.*

*I spent my childhood in a home with busy, achieving,
ministering people. One of my mother's favorite phrases was:
"Make every minute sixty seconds worth of distance run."*

And now as I lay hour after day after week after month in total stillness, running no distance . . . guilt struck my child-heart with such fearsome, consistent blows that I could not even cry out. Only deep within, the child-voice howled in torture.

I was consumed with self-hatred until I took the time and effort to understand the little girl still within me, the little girl wanting to obey her mother. Genuine growth, I began to perceive, means having the courage and confidence to tread new paths, and in the process, leave old ones behind.

Mother's dictum worked for her. It had worked for me for many years. It was no longer relevant. I ceased being victim to my guilt. I ceased disclaiming the child huddling in fear within me. Instead I claimed the child's terror as realistic . . . and comforted it as I strove to release that part of my past and turn my focus toward a new way to live. I made the choice not to turn against that child . . . but to face the need for change with all the kindness I would muster for Billy and Ronnie . . . and give the child time to grow with the same grace I would offer to my sons.

8. I WILL REJOICE IN THE PERSON I AM BECOMING . . . BECAUSE OF GOD'S REDEMPTION. I owe the person I am today to this illness. Had I remained the competent, active professional, I would have never known the inner Ruth. That would have been my loss. She is worth knowing well.

Also, today, I am stronger in courage, wiser in faith, more indestructible under attack. Oddly, I am more independent. Although I am totally dependent on medication and the care of my husband and sons, even to stay alive, I am more independent in spirit than before.

I have become a different person in vital areas. I have a different perspective. I have a different level of patience, sympathy, tolerance, compassion. All of this is part of growth. Painful growth forced upon me. But good growth, and I wear my battle scars proudly!

I don't know why this happened. I can be at peace without the answer. I have pleasant, poignant memories of the active life, but I also know there is joy in the slow, silent life. I live a different pace; I use different skills; I give through different channels. But that is not bad. Just different. I rejoice in the person-ever-becoming . . . the person created in the fiery furnace of my own personal pain.

16
Looking for Joy

We all easily admit that compassionate caring is needed from people on the outside. I believe it is as necessary a gift to oneself. Perhaps more so.

Many of my friends at the university were performers. Some that I knew best were incredibly talented. They often received standing ovations, curtain calls, lavish adulation from their audiences. But when they returned to their dressing rooms, I watched them sink into the depths of despair.

The applause from the audience was fleeting. What they needed most was *approval from the inside*. They never heard themselves say: "You did well."

Once after receiving an award, I was being "properly modest" as I received congratulations from a friend, and was shocked when he said: "Ruth, why don't you *accept* the joy? *You did it!*"

I have always remembered that. I would have been jumping up and down shouting "hosannahs" had one of my friends won that award. I felt free to give commendation to another. I began to understand that I should also be free in giving commendation to self. And, perhaps, I needed it more from self than any other.

Involved also in learning to "love self" was the determination to begin to *listen* to self. I was startled to realize how effectively I had tuned my inner voice *out*. Always wanting to please,

I had listened to exterior voices and complied. I had lived from *the outside in.*

This "tuning in" was a difficult procedure.

I had stopped listening to self for so long that my own voice had grown almost inaudible. I could barely hear it. I had to urge it to speak at all.

And yet, in that self-voice lay the "life-changing-wisdom" needed for this illness. My doctor had said it had to come from deep inside me. He was right.

When I understood my need for self-friendship, I knew that "alarm clocks" would be unnecessary. Inside, I had always known where my "parameters" lay. The problems had occurred because I had refused to listen to my inner voice.

And so I began to try.

When I was too weak to make it down the hall, I lay down on the carpet to wait for strength. When I tried to type and weakness overwhelmed, I lay in the floor by the typewriter. When the family was in the kitchen and I wanted to be with them, I lay on the floor or they laid me on the cabinet.

Inside, *I* knew how far I could walk; how long I could type; *if* I could sit up. And when I listened to the inner voice, instead of focusing on will power, I found that I *could* live inside the limited parameters. Gradually, my inner friend, who whispered in the beginning, grew in confidence to speak with definite authority.

Involved also in learning to love self was acceptance of my moods. I had enjoyed being a victim of whatever "came over me." "I just couldn't help the sadness," I wrote one day, "and so I cried until I was ill."

Well, I couldn't help *the sadness* . . . but I could *choose* response to the sadness. It is all wrapped up in focus.

I can *choose,* instead, to rejoice in the redbirds filling the tree outside my window. I can *choose* to think of my three men's current activities and pace in the excitement (vicariously) with them. I can *choose* to turn "The Hallelujah Chorus" recordings on fortissimo . . . and if I do any of these things, if tears crop up, they spring upwards in joy. One simply cannot be sad when enveloped in the majesty of Handel's great music.

There are times, however, when I can't play "The Hallelujah Chorus" fortissimo. Perhaps because it is in the middle of the night and everyone else is sleeping. Perhaps I simply *will not* move at the moment. There are no redbirds. I don't even *know* what my three men are doing.

And the tears slide. My heart bulges. I mourn.

In the beginning, I would chastise myself unmercifully for not *choosing* to be cheerful. I finally learned to *shut up* the strident voice dealing in "what should be" . . . and listen carefully to the wounded soul inside grieving over "what is." For I learned that courage is all well and good, but it is only a partial answer.

One must mourn. And it does not complete itself in the first week after the carousel dies. It goes on. For years.

Mourning is a slow, dark, wordless process. But it is vital if healing is to come.

Just as acceptance of the blow takes time to filter through all the vulnerable, sensitive tissues of the subconscious, so healing continues for a long period in many levels of the spirit. Mourning is an essential part of getting well. And if I would be a friend to self, I would understand when it is time for "The Hallelujah Chorus" . . . and when it is time to mourn.

Now, after a tearful bout of sorrow, I try to discover the specific torture point that was draining pent-up pain. Now that the abscess is emptied, it can heal. And I revel in the warmth of returning wholeness.

There are, of course, times when I simply give in to grieving over the injustice. Although futile, it is human. And I strive for forgiveness.

Forgiveness.

That is a gift I have truly tried to give to self . . . for the first time in my life. All the kind, thoughtful things I would do for my husband, my children . . . all the loving, supportive forgiveness I would offer them, I offer myself.

There are times when I actually say aloud to the sobbing-child-inside: "I know. I understand. Remember, I was there too. I know the fear, the unrelenting terror of life stripped of all you had planned for, trusted in. I know.

"But it will be all right. I promise. It will be all right."

156 / M<small>Y</small> G<small>OD</small>, M<small>Y</small> G<small>OD</small>!

And strange as it may seem, the calm, steady adult voice (speaking with gentle strength) comforts me.

I have tried to become such a friend-to-self that I know when I should speak . . . when I should be silent . . . when I should make demands. For there are times when I need to be left alone to think things through logically. There are other times when I need assertive decision: "All right. Enough of that." And I, the adult, choose to turn my focus to other things.

My brother once asked: "How do you keep from being afraid when you are in this house by yourself so much?"

I answered: "I choose not to be."

He blinked. "You mean . . . just like that?"

I grinned at his surprise to my quick, almost vehement, answer.

It is that simple. It is also that complex.

Because sometimes the choice has to be made every hour. Sometimes every minute. But it *is* still a choice.

My friend, Vickie, made me an adorable ceramic doll.

Bill brought her in at night and I could not see her well in the dimly lit room. But the next morning, I went into the living room and lay on the floor in front of her.

She had on a blue dress; her head drooped; her eyes were downcast.

After a moment, I said: "Hello, little girl. I'm glad you came to live with me."

I reached out to her.

"But are you sad? If you are, we should be very good friends because, you see, I know all about sadness."

I looked her over carefully.

And then I touched her hand and said aloud: "But look! Here is a yellow butterfly on your hand. What you must learn is to focus your mind on the beauty of God's world . . . and when you do . . . you'll find, to your amazement, that the sadness will slip away."

There was a sound in the doorway and I turned to see Bill standing there listening to my talking to the doll. There were tears in his eyes.

That noon he brought me a butterfly in a frame. Friends were told the experiences and now my house is ablaze with butterflies . . . each a symbol of love, of caring . . . each a symbol to remind me to keep my focus on loveliness . . . no matter how alone are my days.

It is true!

I look for the *joy* in everything.

When I take a bath, I literally *revel* in the tingle of muscles relaxing in the steaming whirlpool of bubbles.

When I drink hot cocoa or eat a banana split, I *savor* each drop, each bite for the sensory pleasure that it gives.

When I wear flannel pajamas (now my favorite of all clothing), I snuggle in their softness and caress the clinging warmth.

Little things.

And the big things . . . like Ronnie whom I overheard one day talking with a high school chum. The topic was one of my plays currently playing in a dinner theater in Denver.

Brian said: "I bet it makes her sad not to get to see her own play."

Ron responded: "I guess. She never says. But I think it's okay because . . . you see, she chose to live this way for me!"

My heart caught on a gasp of gratitude. He understood his worth.

Like Billy who introduced me to a new girl friend with the words: "My mom turns the world on with her smile." I could not contain the tears.

Like Bill. I sometimes apologize for "turning out like I did" and he, the Ph.D. in communication skills, assures me that I "turned out better than dreams." When I challenge the stupidity of such a statement, he says seriously: "But it's true. I miss your physical hand-holding in the race . . . but we are ever together. I think your thoughts. I laugh your laugh. No matter where I am, no matter how busy is my mind and body, *you* are there. The unit is indissoluble." And I know he cherishes the simple love-gift that is the only one I now can give: me.

The big things.

Frost wrote:

Two roads diverged in a wood
And I,
I took the one less traveled by,
And that has made all the difference.

That certainly is true in building a new world. One stands at a Y . . . and chooses the geographical location for his creation.

Will it be in the valley or in the mountains?

Will it be in the abyss of self-pity and whining or on the peak of gratitude and giving?

When you turn from a dead life-carousel, you will find:

"Two roads diverged in a wood . . ." and you must make your choice. And that one decision will make all the difference.

Another change I had known from the beginning that would have to be made was the redefining of life. Slowly I was able to do that.

I had defined life in the exterior realm of doing.

I now defined it in the interior realm of being.

I had lived from the outside in.

I changed to live from the inside out.

Life was no longer the "God-Service-Way."

Life was now the "God-Companioned-Way."

This was an important brick in the building of a new world.

I had understood, from the first moments of discussing the "little old lady" that it would mean a total reassessment of values.

This task was filled with knife-points. Everytime I tried to pick up a piece for the new construction, it would be surfaced with slashing blades.

There were times the old hierarchy rose up from the past as if to choke me. I wanted to scream aloud and batter with my fists at the immovable illness. *"It isn't worth it!"* I would cry. *"Nothing can possibly be worth all this!"*

But I kept trying. Working in, between, around the torture-blades I kept trying.

And gradually brick began to top brick and I could see the beginnings of a new edifice of values. Gradually out of the great black cold, a warm light was blown into my mind, a luminous vibration, a surety greater than sorrow or privation or a dead carousel.

There is no point in enumerating at length. One example will clarify.

I have always been an articulate speaker—in demand for all kinds of public speaking occasions to share my "wisdom." That service was of high value in my hierarchy.

In a split second of time, it was gone. Not only was I not speaking for conventions, I found I often did not have the strength to talk at all. I would lie very still, very quietly until one of my men would come in.

Since speaking was beyond my ability, I developed a clue to communication. I would whisper weakly: "I can listen."

It's a favorite teasing phrase in our house.

"I can listen."

This clues them into the fact that I can *not* respond with my voice, but I want to respond with my eyes that can love . . . with my heart that can rejoice over their happinesses . . . and can sadden over their disappointments . . . with my soul that can pray.

They tease me, these men, but they know it is the only gift I can give at those times . . . and it isn't a very astounding, dazzling, exciting gift . . . not really . . .

But as we have lived through these months and years, I have pondered . . . and I have decided that, perhaps, "I can listen" may be *the* most valuable gift possible.

Were I well and strong, I would be terribly involved in declaring how things *should be.*

Weakened, I listen carefully to *what is.*

And in forgetting *should be* . . . and hand-holding, heart-sharing in *what is,* we are *together* as we face life realistically.

I sometimes wonder if that is not what Jesus meant when He said: "Love one another."

Did He not mean, in a sense, *"Listen* to one another!"?

For so often, in accepting the destruction of the old world, the scream that has ripped from my heart has been: *Won't somebody listen to what it's like to be me in these circumstances? Please, somebody, listen, imagine . . . care!*

Love-lined, accepting listening is a love-gift. It may be of greater value than reams of profound speaking.

An important brick laid in my new world construction. And there are others.

Being, as Jesus told Mary so long ago, is a love-gift. He said it was "the better part."

And so . . . I have chosen to be the simple quiet essence of Ruth inside "limited parameters" so two growing youth can have a mother . . . so that skinny blond I married can have a wife.

In the "old world", I gave them the gifts of wheeling vivacity, eloquent lectures, military-like efficiency, myriad-career competencies, jumping-up-and-down enthusiasm, barefoot-singing laughter.

In the new world, I give the gift of release because I want them to be free . . . even of me. I give the gift of listening because I am not strong enough to deal with "should be." I give the gift of joy because I choose to focus on the glory and wonder splashing pell-mell all about me, dazzling skyrockets of pure happiness . . . even in life-less-than-ideal.

Bill bought me a miniature Raggedy Andy sitting in his own wicker chair the other day. It filled me with total delight. I showed it to Ron and bubbled about its wonder. I said: "I just look and look and look at it. It makes me laugh in its cheerfulness."

Ron ruffled my hair in his special way and said: "What a strange lady you are! It takes the smallest things to make you happy!"

I reached up to kiss him and found tears in his eyes. "You are really special," he said. And I wept in his arms.

Later I wrote in my journal:

To build a new world is a pretty phrase. But it takes a long, long, time to make it come true.

It isn't faith that held me steady for this long rebuilding. It's more than faith. I had faith when I was a little girl. I had faith when I wrote my credo on the flyleaf of my Bible in St. Luke's Hospital in 1966. Now I've proven God's Presence. I've proven God's redemption. No. It isn't faith enabling me to begin a new world.

It is fact.

17

Friendly Persuasion

As the years rolled by, my friends became more and more intrigued with the *why* of my illness. The discomfort they had felt in the beginning had now given way to dusty habit. My dilemma was as normal to them now as the sun rising. And so it began to feed intellectual discussions.

During this period I was deluged with the explanations my friends had formulated as to why my world had been blasted. And in their explanations were their attempts to persuade me to consider pat answers to the Why? of my suffering.

One of the explanations was: *Because God loves you so much.* I remember one person's writing me, in awe, "For all you have gone through, *God must really love you!*"

It made no sense to me whatsoever. I knew that line of reasoning grew out of the school of thought that teaches that earthly suffering gives one greater merit in the beyond. But if that were true, then when God chose one (like me) for unusual suffering, did that not indicate favoritism? If so, I would prefer, at the moment, to be one of the *less* favored!

No. I could not believe that God had chosen me for unusual pain because He loved me more than others. I believe He loves all children equally. "The rain falls on the just and the unjust." Natural law felled me as it has felled others, while many have been untouched by its tornadoes and experienced only its sun-

161

shine. Such is part and parcel of living within a world governed by natural law.

Others wrote that *the illness was all part of a plan whose purpose I had no right to know.* I recognized the roots of this argument in the doctrine of predestination and, at certain moments, it was comforting to snuggle in. But when I was thinking clearly, I could not accept it. If there were a purpose in God's allowing me to achieve a meaningful life of giving to others, only to lose it, why would He not reveal that purpose to *me?*

Probably the explanation offered most consistently was that *through suffering, others could learn life's lessons.* I was their substitute. These are the ones who wrote prolific letters of gratitude for all I was doing for *them.*

But that theory offered no explanation I could find reasonable. In the first place, why was I chosen as the substitute? And where was *my* substitute?

In the second place, what would happen when tragedy struck these friends of mine? Would that not annihilate their theory of substitution? No. It had no substance and vanished like morning mist.

Others suggested it was just "fate." One of my kindest friends wrote me, "When your time comes for suffering, you just have to accept it." I was astonished because I could not believe "fate" could coexist with a loving God who participated in the lives of His children. Yet, I discovered that many sincere Christians are convinced that "fate" is the answer.

I was not. I could not believe that God plays dolls with His children until He becomes weary, and then, like an angry child, whams the life out of them. Such caprice is inconsistent with my understanding of the character of the Almighty.

And then there was *the theory of good and evil.* Along with this came *the concept of balances:* Life is equalled out between happiness and sorrow, good and evil, illness and health.

I would often read these letters and wonder if, for every time I had laughed in my first world, I now had to pay with as many tears . . . I had to descend a certain number of degrees into hell for each moment of glory . . . I had to be placed on the torture rack for every moment I had flitted on the mountain peaks.

As my mind worked it through, I could not accept it. It seemed more pagan than Christian. Isn't that what the primitive tribes believed when they threw innocent babies into fiery furnaces to appease their gods?

But we must struggle with the problem of evil in our world. Twenty centuries of Christian scholars have studied it with no complete answer. Certainly I do not have one. My only answer is that focusing on the presence of evil leads to pessimism, hopelessness, and even fatalism.

I wrote in my journal:

The best solution I can now find can be expressed in this analogy. When the children were little, our next-door neighbor was a lady who despised children, dogs, and noise. All three existed often in our back yard. When the neighbor became especially irritated, she would come to the fence in the back yard for attack. At such times my tiny sons did not try to work out a solution with her. Instead, they stayed in close contact with their mother (just inside the kitchen door). And when the irritated woman stormed into the yard, the little boys simply called out, "Mother!" and went back to their play.

I, who was the same size, age, and intelligence as the lady, could then try to resolve the problem. But the battle was mine, not my children's. They were not wise enough. They had to trust that battle to me.

In thinking through this problem with evil, I realize that I am not big enough, strong enough, wise enough to meet the Devil's attacks. So it seems to me that my role is to stay close to my Heavenly Father. When attacked, I simply call: "Dear God!" . . . and He comes to the "fence" to deal with the attacker.

It would be as ludicrous for me to try to pit my puny resources against Satan as it would have been for Billy and Ronnie to have tried to reason with the neighbor. Just as they were not equal to interchange with her, so am I not equal to the powers of evil. But I have "close contact" with One who is. And so I will simply call for His help . . . and trust Him to work it all out.

My academic friends, of course, offered *materialism*. Some of my colleagues did admit there was a Supreme Being, but they felt my illness was only further proof that the "reins of the universe are tangled in the frantic hands of God."

At the university we had had many debates as to whether God was omnipotent or helpless as a paper tiger. There was a "Starter Force" in the universe, many admitted, but man was only higher than the animals in the sense that he does have choice. In their minds the "Starter Force" was impotent in dealing with the chaos caused by those choices. So, many of my university colleagues only felt pity for God . . . and for me who believed Him omnipotent.

They now wrote asking me to recant my position. I could not. If God is intelligent enough to be the "Starter Force" of the universe, He is certainly intelligent enough to guide and control it.

"So why did He not control your pituitary gland?" they asked. And my answer was: "He is in control so that *nothing* *ir*redeemable can or will occur. *This* can be redeemed!" How? I had not the faintest notion. But I was determined to *believe* He stood the Redeemer God!

Ultimately I looked at my problem in the light of plain common sense. My mother was forty-four when I was born. She had an abdominal tumor. Under the best of conditions, defective babies are often born to older mothers. I was born with a sluggish pituitary gland that finally ceased to function altogether.

But it was not God's will that illness blast my life at age thirty-nine!

I have studied the Bible intensely. I have read many learned theologians. I have almost memorized the Gospels. And I have found no pat answer to the why. But I *have* found God incarnate in human history.

As I read the Gospels, I find Jesus accepting human existence unequivocally. He accepted evil and suffering as part of this world. He wasted no time agonizing over the gaping wound of grief and torment in creation. He did not ask *who* was to blame. He did not ask *why* it was fact.

Instead, he bypassed all of that and accepted the wound in creation as the mystery of existence. He devoted His life to giving loving compassion such as the world has never seen . . .

lavish caring, sharing such as the world has never known.

In spite of all the Pharisees tried to do, the crowds read in Jesus' eyes God's love for them in their troubles and they flocked to Him. And He said: "Blessed are the pure in heart, for they shall see God. . . . Blessed are they that mourn for they shall be comforted. . . . Blessed are the poor in spirit for they shall inherit the Kingdom of heaven."

No explanation of suffering in the Gospels, then—just Jesus, God's Son in a suffering world.

No pat answers to illuminate pain and suffering in the Gospels—just Jesus, God's Incarnate Love beautifully and totally illuminated.

I wrote in my journal:

The more I study Jesus, the more I believe that the why that has so plagued my soul is irrelevant. Perhaps I can find no answer for it because there is no answer for it. More, perhaps, I can find no answer for it because the answer is not needed.

He accepted human sorrow in this world as a fact. He spent no time on questions. He moved quickly into meeting it with life.

After arriving at these conclusions, I made another entry in my journal:

So. Now I write these items as part of my credo.

1. LIFE IS GOING TO GO ON. There are three men depending on me. Whatever happens, the streams of life must flow on through me, in me, with me. Defeat is never to be a possibility for consideration. Depression has no place in my life. I will find a happy, contributing way to live for three men.

2. GOD IS WITH ME. Within the laws of the natural order, pituitary glands stop working just as within the laws of free choice, Mike can walk away to divorce Kenna. Some things happen because we belong to human society. But God's will is for life to be lived most abundantly. At this moment, mine cannot reach that fullness and He weeps with me. He holds my hand and cares. But because He is a Redeemer God, He will enable me to build a new world where the abundant life is a possibility, if I allow. I will allow.

3. DEATH IS ONLY A DOOR TO THE LARGER LIFE.

There is no fear. To love life, one must also love death because death is life's fulfillment. Those who see only life's phenomena cling to life like a miser clings to a debased currency, which is, in the end, worthless. Clinging to life is not loving life. Loving life is accepting its rhythms and moving in step with them. What is begun here will be completed there. So nothing is ever lost out of God's care.

More and more, as I struggled in new world-building, I began to find a realistic, sensible philosophy.

I wrote in my journal:

I am learning acceptance. Whatever is, is. I can't change it. Weeping, wondering, wishing has no place in my life. The thing to do now is the very best I can IN THESE CIRCUMSTANCES and leave the rest to God.

I know so much of my life seems waste as I totter alone up and down these hallways. But I refuse to believe it. If life gave opportunity for me to be an active professional in the midst of people, then I should be the very best active professional I could be. By the same token, if life is offering me the opportunity to be a "little old lady" inside four walls, then let me determine to be the best little old lady possible!

Don't fight what is, Ruth. Some questions have no answers; there is mystery in dealing with the Infinite God. So put your hand in His hand and get on with life. You can sing the Lord's song inside four walls . . . if you choose to!

I found this poem and I like it:

Oh, I have heard a golden trumpet blowing
Under the night. Another warmth than blood
Has coursed, though briefly, through my intricate veins.
Some sky is in my breast where swings a hawk
Intemperate for immoralities
And unpersuaded by the show of death
I am content with what I cannot prove.

—William Alexander Percy

And, so, tonight, as I sit here in my flannel pajamas alone, I have a sense of peace. I have read these many letters, written by my *"friendly persuaders." I have formed my own answer. It calls for action; it challenges me to go on . . . even now. I have refused to believe in a helpless God, a punishing God, a "play-favorites" God, or a God who blindfolds me.*

I have peace tonight because I am in alliance with the Almighty God who is omnipotent, but who, nonetheless, respects me. Now there is an incredible thought. God and I have mutual respect and love.

Incredible, it may seem. Truth, I assert it to be.

And that takes the tension out of my cry that so often rises in sheer panic: *Life isn't supposed to be like this!* I am walking this road with God. That is the one answer I know and accept.

Oh, the process is far from complete. Some days are unbearably painful; some moments I feel so hollow I am afraid I may break; some nights I walk the hallways warily. The least little jostle might shatter me . . . not physically . . . emotionally. I often feel I am on an abandoned trestle of rotting planks pursued by an illness that wants to break me to bits.

But the power of those torture-times is not as great now. I have a weapon to fight them—a weapon won in fearful, faithful battle—an increasing proving of the Redeemer God *with*.

I am not a fan of Albert Camus. Yet, in the midst of all the various explanations presented to me, he gave one of the most helpful:

> Losing a loved (world), uncertainty about what we are, these are deprivations that give rise to our worst suffering. We may be idealistic, but we need what is tangible. It is by the presence of persons and things that we believe we recognize certainty. And though we may not like it, at least we live with this necessity.
>
> But the astonishing . . . thing is that these deprivations bring us the cure at the same time that they give rise to pain. Once we have accepted the fact of loss, we understand that the loved one obstructed a whole corner of the possible, pure now as a sky washed by rain. Freedom emerges from weariness. To be happy is to stop. Free, we seek anew, enriched by pain. And the perpetual impulse forward always falls back again to gather new strength. The fall is brutal, but we set out again.

After the quote, I wrote:

I've been sitting here trying to think it through. He is right. He is right. It's just that it all hurts so much and requires so much courage to face . . . that I want to deny it. But he is right. What was not possible in the old world is possible now.

An important example is time for my three men. I am always here for them now. I can share everything with them now. And although I tried to be available when needed in the old world, I wasn't always. They didn't always come first. Now they can. And that is one way that when I "have accepted the fact of loss, (I) understand that the loved (world) obstructed a whole corner of the possible, pure now as a sky washed by rain. Freedom emerges . . . Free, (I) seek anew, enriched by pain. . . ."

Yes, I think I understand what he is saying and I think he is right. I will build a new world, one I could have never known had the old one not been taken away. There will be, in that new world, relationships and adventures, possibilities and potentials, that were not available before. So although I did not wish that "corner of my world" to be "pure as sky washed by rain," it is . . . and in that purity does lie opportunity for joyful things, happy experiences . . . a new world that could not have existed before.

Camus didn't know, of course, but he was really saying: He is a Redeemer God always with His beloved child.

I wish I could tell Camus. I'm sorry he never knew.

18

Address the
Mystery With Life

The Gospels tell me Jesus accepted human sorrow in this world as a fact. He spent no time on questions. He moved quickly into meeting reality with life itself.

That is what I knew I must do.

I chose this as the first erected timber of a new world. I will bypass the why . . . and ask how the Redeemer God and I can make creative use . . . now?

I began to try it.

When I would awake in the morning, I would check strength levels and then ask: "Lord, how can You and I find creative use of 'this much' today?" And whatever answer came to mind, I would set myself about it.

If the answer was that I could not move from the bed that day, I bypassed *why* . . . and asked *how* . . . and the answer would always be: *pray*. Without moving a muscle, I could open a prayer channel for the beloved people of my life in the detail that they needed.

In the whoosh and activity of life, one always promises: "I'll pray for you." One wants to. Plans to. Would like to. But there isn't time.

Well . . . I had time.

And so I prayed.

When the strength level was such that I could go to the

typewriter, I would work as long as possible. When my inner voice said: "Enough," I lay on the floor hoping for a second wind. If it came, I got back in the chair and typed again. If it did not, I finally would arise and totter into the bed and relax in what is.

Now.

You do understand that I am writing the results of *years* of work. It sounds so glib. It sounds so simple. It sounds so blithe.

It was none of these things.

It was hideous.

I did not want to lie in bed. Even to pray. I wanted to be *up* running around the block.

When I got to the typewriter, I never wanted to stop. And when I did give in, I didn't want to relax in *what is.* I wanted to be angry and scream and throw things at *what is!*

Sometimes I did.

Sometimes I didn't.

I just kept working at it.

Trying. Failing. Forgiving. Trying again.

But more and more, I was completely bypassing the *why.* More and more, my life was dominated by *how.*

To spotlight before me my focal point, I ordered large wooden letters spelling out the word HOW. I arranged them to stand across my window sill. Whenever I opened my eyes, H-O-W pulled me to its question and the searing inner question of W-H-Y slid into oblivion.

Bill began to utilize the concept in his teaching.

In an adult seminar in discipling, he told the story of my wooden letters and their meaning. Later, someone in the class left a beautiful macramé cross on his desk. In the middle of the crossbeams was the large wooden letter H. The wooden letters on the two sides of the horizontal beam spelled: WHO. The wooden letters on the bottom of the vertical beam spelled: HOW.

In his discussion with the group, Bill had made the point that we need not know *why* when we know *who* for He will show *how* . . . and we can address the mystery of suffering *with life.*

With the cross was a note of gratitude to Bill for the concept. It was unsigned.

Bill placed the cross on the wall of his office. He uses its symbols in counseling almost every day of his ministry. And when Billy assumed his position as full-time minister of youth, he also bought large wooden letters H-O-W to put in his office to assist him in counseling teens who are caught in the web of despair.

Many suffering people come to those offices wanting to ponder upon, brood over, ask why they must suffer. Ultimately, we have to concede mystery, bypass the why, and make ourselves instruments for the alleviation of the suffering.

I can remember times when loneliness would almost strangle me. I would feel such a *need* for someone to reach out to me . . . for someone to say *words* of caring, sharing, support. Instead of lingering in my own mystery of why I had to be lonely and needy, I would go to the typewriter and write someone *the words I so deeply wanted someone to say to me!*

Since I so personally understood how much love and compassion is needed in the midst of human sorrow, I could use that knowledge to try to become an instrument of love and compassion to alleviate the pain and suffering of others. This was an important HOW!

I would address the mystery with life.

Bill began a full-scale drama program in Denver. He needed quality religious plays. There were only a few.

In my later professional life, I had concentrated my writing on books. Though I had written everything—Sunday school curriculum from nursery age to goldenagers, Vacation Bible school curriculum, movie scripts, television scripts, short stories, poetry, essays, columns, readings, skits, and plays—books had been my greatest love. And so in ranking priorities, I had placed a published book a year as fulfillment in my life-arena.

Of course, I hadn't held to that schedule. The few plays I had written in college were born out of my own enthusiasms, and I moved on to other enthusiasms with little thought to what had been created.

Now I wondered. Could this be a way of God's making creative use out of the academic, experiential expertise . . . *even now?* I had no idea if I would be strong enough.

And so I asked God: *How?*

And this is what we worked out.

When it was essential, I would lie "very still" while the brain created. No matter how frozen the body, the brain could jump and spin and whirl and dance with all the abandon of the old world. So I trained myself to think it all through: the structure, the movement, the dialogue.

And then, on those days when there was strength, I could sit at the typewriter and it would flow through my fingers, full-birthed. Often it did not have to be retyped.

And so *Little Christmas* was born. And then the play based on the work of fiction I love most, Eugenia Price's *The Beloved Invader.*

All of this was painstakingly slow. The body remained in severe difficulty. Medications had to be changed. Life was precarious. But keeping my eyes on those wooden letters on my window sill, I kept asking HOW? . . . and plodding along.

I remember one summer day. In the mail was an alumni paper. I opened it listlessly and scanned its pages. Suddenly I saw my name and perked up.

It was contained in an article detailing the experience of the writer at a performance of *The Beloved Invader.* The author said he had been trapped into going by the cousin he was visiting. He *hated* religious plays but was being a "good sport." He had not known the playwright's name until the first intermission. Shocked, he told his companion that he had gone to graduate school with me.

When he learned of my illness, he said, "I was subdued as the second act began . . . I remembered that young woman. She was on top then. She was respected, envied, even hated for her perceptive mind, the quality of her work. But of course, she could *be* religious! She had everything going her way! Now she didn't. But she still found a way to use that inimitably creative mind for her God."

I remembered him. I was pleased to know he remembered me.

He was lavish in his praise of the play. Although he admitted his distaste for religious plays, he felt this was written with "the finesse of Neil Simon." And then he concluded: "I keep thinking of that brilliant energetic young woman in my classes, now in a lifetime illness, who is still finding ways to use that inimitably creative mind. She said in her play: 'It is the way of the Redeemer God.' I never believed there was a God, but now I sort-of-hope there is. And if there is, I hope He is *that kind.*"

I was flattered by his praise. I enjoyed his superlatives. But I got lost in remembering that "energetic young woman" . . . and the sorrow for that lost world whammed me with vigor.

I went to bed with a troubled heart.

Bill was in Vail, Colorado, directing this same play for an International Singles' Retreat. After the performance, he called me and after a few bits of information, he gave the phone to a young man who had been my counselee for the four years of his college life.

Lewis said: "Mrs. Vaughn, I love you. I just saw your play. I felt and heard you in every line. In it is all the philosophy you used to shape my life."

After I hung up the phone, I lay in the dark remembering that young, seeking freshman who had hurtled himself into my world . . . into my life and followed my directives in even the most personal areas of his development.

He had truly been *my kid!*

He had played Creon when I directed *Antigone.* He had *become* Mark Twain in his senior speech recital. He had been my constant delight in writing classes. The essays he spun cupped a wry humorous satire that made me laugh even as I red-penciled *all* his spelling errors.

He had carried my books to class. He had raced me across campus, having the grace to allow me to win. He had brought me hamburgers when I worked through a meal. And he asked my advice on dating, love, marriage, priorities, Christian living . . . and whatever else came into his mind.

For four years, from freshman to senior, he had paced with me. I was his academic counselor, his communication counselor, his personal counselor.

And when he graduated and went out to become a successful competent adult, he wrote me a note. He outlined all the things he had accomplished in his college years. And then he concluded succinctly: "Because of you."

Now it was over.

Lewis said on the phone: "In (your play) is all the philosophy you used to shape my life."

I would never "shape" a life like that again.

I would never know activity like that again.

I would never be of God-use like that again.

I finally fell into a restless sleep.

I dreamed I was back on campus. Three of my students were talking together. There was Lewis . . . now a hospital administrator; Debbie . . . now a youth magazine editor; Sue . . . now "starring" in *The Beloved Invader.*

Those three beloved students were chatting with animation, and my heart swelled with dreams for them, love for them . . . but they didn't see me. I could not join their laughter, I could not share their vivacity. I could not participate in their verbal banter . . . because I no longer had the strength to teach in college!

In my dream, I turned to God and said: *I can't ever work for You like that again. I can't ever do any of those things again!*

My heart squirmed with pain.

Don't you see what has happened? I cried. *I can't ever be of God-use . . . with my hands and feet, with my enthusiasm and exuberance, with my dynamism and jumping joy! O God! Dear God! That has to be a waste! That has to be a waste!*

I sagged into a heavy heap, much like a ragged, spilled-out grain sack.

How can You possibly redeem such loss?

And . . . in my dream God said: "But don't you think an *'inimitably creative mind'* could be a God-tool?"

I woke up . . . laughing.

Just as I had laughed when I read the article where the writer had used the phrase "inimitably creative mind" twice. Both God and I knew how absurd that was . . . we had laughed together and I had dismissed it.

Now, with His infinite humor, He used the phrase in an earnestness that demanded from me an answer.

"Don't you think an 'inimitably creative mind" could be a God-tool?"

Well. Perhaps.

I had always adored writing. Some of my first memories were my attempts at poetry and songs to sing to God in my mulberry tree. Somehow I wanted them to be original . . . things shared only between my heart and God's. Sunday school poetry, Sunday school songs had no place in my mulberry tree. Only free expression written in scrawling pencil on Red Chief tablets.

Always an avid reader, I had especially responded to *Emily of New Moon.* I had memorized the part where she talked about her need to write. "Tell me this," she had been challenged, "if you knew that you would be poor as a church mouse all your life—if you knew you'd never have a line published—would you still go on writing—would you?"

Emily had been as disdainful as I. What on *earth* did money and publishing have to do with writing? One wrote because . . . because . . . as she said: "I can't help it . . . I've just got to."

"Oh—then, I'd waste my breath giving advice at all. If it's in you to climb you must—there are those who must lift their eyes to the hills—they can't breathe properly in the valleys . . . Go on—climb!"

I'd quoted that admonition to myself a million times through my life. When all the other activities of my life crowded in so that it seemed wise to relegate writing to a miniscule slot, I would remember those words. And sighing with joy in the release of that freedom, I would carve out a chunk in my busy schedule for the glory of climbing through the magic of written words.

"Don't you think 'an inimitably creative mind" can be a God-tool?" The body lay still . . . but the mind could *climb* . . . *climb* . . . *soar* . . . even as the Catskill eagle.

Could I? My heart quaked at the whole concept.

I reached for Morris West's book, *The Shoes of the Fisherman.* I had marked a paragraph in it the day before. I wanted to reread it.

I opened to the page.

It costs so much to be a full human being that there are very few who have the enlightenment or the courage to pay the price . . . One has to abandon altogether the search for security, and reach out to the risk of living with both arms. One has to embrace the world like a lover. One has to accept pain as a condition of existence. One has to court doubt and darkness as the cost of knowing. One needs a will stubborn in conflict, but apt always to total acceptance of every consequence of living and dying.

The image was clear before me, beckoning me *to build a new world.* I remembered other journal writings where I asserted that I would "build for the second half of my life much as I built for the first: creatively, with my whole heart."

"One has to accept pain as a condition of existence." Bypass the *why*; move on to the *how* . . .

"One has to court doubt and darkness as the cost of knowing." Could writing be a means of still actively participating in the world? There was doubt in my mind . . . there was darkness on the horizon so I could not see the answer . . . but I would dare.

I would address the mystery of suffering *with life* in every way I could discover. Perhaps this was of God.

I began playwriting as a major *how* for me.

The need for love is universal. In our mass, computerized society, there seems to be less and less of it. We rush about playing roles, with little time to really give or receive love.

My husband wrote in a book on the need for small groups:

Even in the warmest, friendliest church, we don our nicest clothes, our most pleasing smiles, and our best cultivated manners. We respond to greetings that we are "fine," "the weather is beautiful," and the children are all "well." It is only in the eyes that the perceptive listener might see pain burning like twin martyr fires and understand the aching, strangling problems of our hearts.

But in our rushing society, even the perceptive cannot often linger to help. There are too many other pressures, too many other calls, too many other demands. So, with a sigh of relief, even the perceptive person scurries away, pretending to believe our lie that "all's right with the world."

In one way, love had been taken from my life when I was placed inside my house-boundaries. I was not only taken from the arena where people gather, but people were asked not to come here.

As my plays began to be performed regularly, love in another form began flooding into my life in veritable waves.

Typical was a letter from an elderly lady:

"I am eighty-six years old and stay alone in my home, take care of myself, drive my own car. I go to church when I can. I went to see your recent play. I was so touched by its message I asked someone who wrote it. They showed me your picture and told me you were ill. I asked for your address because I wanted to write and thank you. . . . Because of the play, I feel as if I know you well. I laughed at your humor. I cried at your portrayal of suffering. I triumphed in your theology. When I looked at your picture, I knew I loved you."

A mother wrote: "I have just returned from your new play. I laughed over many parts—especially that part where the two young mothers did the patter-scene about the unfairness that a baby's first word is "Daddy" when *mothers* do all the work! Would you please let me know—did both your sons do that to you? I am the mother of seven and it happened to me every time!"

A drama professional wrote: "God has given you such a special touch, a glow of His vast creativity, that like embers, you have ignited within me tonight a blaze of joy. Your play is strong, clear, and powerful. It moves well; it holds well; and, most importantly, it communicates."

Soon the fan letters began to transform into loving, personal heart-sharing. Love so complete that one dares to be vulnerable with another can follow only in trust formed by the other's displaying vulnerability, manifesting an understanding of what it's like to be hurt, assuring a lack of judgment of how one responds to deep pain.

Mind must speak to mind. Spirit to spirit.

Incredibly, this happened in my plays.

Following one play, an unknown young woman wrote of her plans to commit suicide. She had already purchased the poison.

The message of the play (based on Romans 8:28) had changed it all.

She wrote: "I didn't know how to tell you this story without telling you everything. I was embarrassed to do that. But I went in the other night and looked at your picture in Dr. Vaughn's office and somehow I knew you'd want to know about my grief. I somehow knew you would understand. I feel you are my friend and will care. So basically I wanted to tell you that I said the 'hardest words' ('Thy will be done') you challenged me within the play and it has changed everything for me. I threw the poison away . . ."

Marital problems, child-rearing problems, bankruptcy problems . . . the trauma of rape, theft, and attempted murder . . . the most personal dilemmas were suddenly coming to my door. These letters often concluded with lines such as these: "Is there hope? Is there a way? I don't know. Could you write me? I feel you could help me deal with this because you know what heartbreak is all about. I would appreciate it if you'd write me. Please, please pray for me."

I had suffered loss of a beloved world.

I had learned to live with life-less-than-ideal.

I knew about pain: emotional, physical, mental.

I knew about injustice, betrayal, rejection, alienation.

And I wrote that knowledge into my plays. And those in the audiences who were confused, bewildered, suffering, mourning identified with me. They felt they could be vulnerable with me. People write me things I am confident they would never verbally say to any other. They trust me, in my isolation, to understand and care in a way they could not trust me were I whirling about as a visible, competent, assured professional.

There is established, in the plays, a heart-bond between me and every person who hurts. They believe that I know *what it's like* to live in a world-gone-crazy. And they reach across the barriers of my house with its invisible "No Visitors" sign and ask me to share their pain.

I can give them no answers to *why*. I can assure them that He is a Redeemer God Who will not waste *anything* . . . when we open ourselves to redemption.

I cannot solve their mystery. I can advise them to follow Jesus' example: *address the mystery with life.*

And they read my words in letters, and listen to them in plays, with an intensity they might not give another. Because I am caught in the mystery myself. I stand on the same ground on which they stand. The cause of the destroyed "old beloved world" may be different, but each "little boat" journeys the same "dark fearful gulf." They allow me, all unseen, to hand-hold with them.

I received this letter recently from a young medical doctor I have never met, but with whom I have gone through one of life's great tragedies via mail. She wrote: "I have just returned home from your beautiful new play. Do you ever feel like Paul writing to his followers? Even though you use drama and he used epistles, the effect is much the same. I went to the play with very negative vibes regarding (personal decision) and as I got into the play, its message hit me right between the eyes. BOING! You've said it to me in letters . . . but in the drama I understand it best: *address the mystery with life.*"

19

Butterflies on Wing

I was trying.

When the mind and body were too weak to move, I tried to serve as a "door-prop" to prayer-channels for those I loved. I would whisper their names and then just hold a silent, unmoving focus upon them, their activities, their needs. No words were said. Often no words were thought. The brain lay as if swamped in molasses. But, by an act of will, I could, even then, serve as a "door-prop" to God.

When the mind would move, but the body would not, I could pray graphically for those in need. Amazing results occurred sometimes. Often I'd feel a strong impression for prayer for one person. Later, a letter would detail how, at that moment, he/she was in great need and felt God come to guide. I participated, thus, in the power of prayer and rejoiced.

When the body could move, my fingers flew in creation . . . and in trying to cope with the towering mountains of mail. Within the mail were letters that all authors receive: asking *how* one writes creatively.

I could not turn those queries off blithely because I had worked hard to earn the academic expertise to share that exact knowledge in a college classroom. That I had done for eight years.

Then, with a wham! bam! shudder! I was placed inside four

walls and the only lecturing that could go on were to my plants and stuffed animals. One particular letter that came with steady regularity in response to all of my books in print, haunted me. They asked me *how* do you do that . . . and, with all my heart, I wanted to tell them!

It was, of course, impossible!

I tried responding with blurred dittos from college classes. It was inadequate and I knew.

One lady I had met in the twelve weeks I was active in the church in Denver, wrote me: "You gave me the dream of writing. And then you went away. You gave me the *want to,* but you could not stay to tell me *how.* What shall I do?"

When Bill came home for lunch, I read her letter and, in tears, shared my frustration. I knew many authors had form letters recommending some textbook which they sent in answer to these queries. That was difficult for me because I had spent years of my life *training to answer that question.*

Now all that academic, as well as experiential, expertise lay dormant inside my brain. How could you call it anything but *waste?*

Bill listened and then suggested that, as I had strength, I simply write out all that I would like to say in response to the questions that kept recurring . . . and through the miracle of Xerox, I could answer in a bit of the depth for which I yearned.

Bill is a wise man. That is what I decided to do.

I bypassed the WHY that I could not teach all this good stuff in college classes and went on to HOW can I put my knowledge in the written word to share with these who ask. I was, thus, addressing the mystery with life.

It worked well. Both I, and my correspondents, were pleased.

As I worked through a stage play for publication, the publisher, knowing my chief credential was book author, asked if I had a manuscript they could consider.

I had some ideas wistfully incubating . . . but a *manuscript* . . . *now?* Wondering how to respond, I had a sudden impulse.

"Would you like to evaluate a manuscript on creative writing?"

There was a swoosh of silence. Now *who* could possibly be interested in publishing a book on creative writing?

But the editor was the epitome of courtesy and asked me to send it along "with no promises because you know this isn't really our interest!" I knew.

Incredibly, it became their interest . . . and the result was the book *Write To Discover Yourself*. I simply could not believe it.

I wrote in my journal:

I wrote this manuscript in defiance of this shattering illness. I didn't write it for publication. I wrote it out of love . . . out of a yearning to share what was inside me in spite of a fragile body . . . out of a determination not to be defeated by unpleasant circumstance.

This manuscript was hammered out in physical pain, in emotional darkness for any kind of future, in such confusion as to WHY . . . But I doggedly bypassed the why and asked how can God and I make creative use of what is in my head . . . now?

And the answer came that I could help Kay, Fran, my own Ron . . . and others who queried me . . . through written words. And so I pounded out chapters on poetry, fiction, and my general philosophy of all writing.

Now, I wrote in wonder, "for this that I created in love for the few, God has opened a door to make available to the masses. I had planned to spend my life teaching the essence of this book to hundreds; now I can share it with thousands. My mind boggles."

I can only gasp: "HE IS a Redeemer God. He does not WASTE . . . anything . . . when we give Him the chance to redeem."

I wrote the incredible account to Genie who had, in her books, laid the foundation on which I had faced this illness and upon which I was now striving to build a superstructure. She understood the miracle and offered to write the introduction to the book.

When she sent it to me, I found within it this concept:

"Ruth Vaughn is, according to all medical wisdom, ill—housebound for the remainder of her life on earth.

"Ruth Vaughn—bound?

"A contradiction. She flies!"

And my tears flooded in gratitude.

She did not know the image of the bird with the broken wing. She did not know my personal determination to build my "nest" in the highlands so that even in the "blackest gorges," there would still be height. She did not know my dream of the "Catskill eagle" who "even if he forever flies within the gorge, that gorge is in the mountains, so that even in his lowest swoop, the mountain eagle is still higher than other birds upon the plain, even though they soar."

It had seemed an impossible dream.

But, all unknowing those personally-meaningful images, Genie wrote: "She flies."

Bill had looked at the book in the city mall long ago: *The Bird With the Broken Wing* and he rushed to the car where he sobbed his despair. Even if I lived, he knew his bird would never fly again.

Later, in Exodus 34:10-11, we had claimed these verses as our own: ". . . this is the contract I am going to make with you. *I will do miracles* such as have never been done before anywhere in all the earth, and all the people . . . shall see the power of the Lord. . . . Your part of the agreement is to obey . . ." (LB)

I had tried to keep my part of that agreement as best I could understand *how*. As always, He had kept His part.

Genie wrote: "She flies."

One of my first breakthroughs in understanding about God and miracles had come that day in the den when I had read to Jill from Thomas Costain's *The Silver Chalice*. It was the time when Christians were huddled in the secret place of the catacombs. They had been informed of Nero's edict that one hundred innocent Christians be slaughtered the next day. When Peter came to them, he shattered their illusion that he would save those doomed Christ-followers from their death. Instead, he reminded them of the steady working of natural law and free choice. Miracles, in the splendid crushing of natural law and free choice, were rare.

Now I went back to Costain's account of this scene. He said that the protagonist of the book, a sculptor named Basil watched the face of the inspired fisherman and he knew that everything

Peter was saying (about the coming mass destruction of Christians by the free choice of the emperor) would come to pass. Luke had prepared him to believe that *a greater miracle* than the delivery of slaves from jail was the *creation of such faith* in the frail hearts of men. *(Italics mine)*

A *greater miracle.*

Could it be that those miracles juggling natural law and free choice are the lesser miracles . . . while the *greater miracles* are those God works within the "frail hearts of men"?

The more I pondered, the more it seemed to be so.

I wrote to my brother about the redemptive event of the book which disproved waste of all that academic, experiential knowledge I had planned to share, in a classroom, for a lifetime. I tiptoed through that "holy ground" with him.

I concluded the letter like this:

"It would be so easy to give in to invalidism. . . .

"It would be so easy to sink in all this weakness and let my brain become mush and my interpersonal contacts rare. . . .

"It would be so easy to dissolve in the loneliness and 'fade away!' But I have determined not to be defeated by a fragile body. The Almighty Sovereign promised: *I will do miracles!*

"I have prayed that the definition of miracle be a revived pituitary gland which would fill my body with racing, riotous, roaring energy. That has not happened.

"So I have daily, often hourly, deliberately opened myself to the 'greater miracle' . . . God with . . . asking Him to enable me to know that the ground on which I stand . . . even the ground of illness that defies all prior-dreams-coming-true . . . on that ground . . . to discover that it is holy ground because He is standing on it with me . . . And because He has promised to do miracles, He will enable me to find creative use of even dream-splintering circumstances . . . and find other dreams filled with splendor beyond even my far-reaching imagination!

"Now *there* is a miracle!

"I now believe that the 'greater miracle' may come when one discovers that although an undesired plateau in life . . . the understanding that dreams (as hung on golden stars for a lifetime) are not going to come true . . . *through His redemption*

. . . *through His presence with.* . . . Those dreams can seed new dreams, can bring new joys, can bring wider ministry, can give birth to a *new world!*

"I sent one of my students a Dollygram when her engagement was broken. On it, I wrote: *'New worlds can be exciting!'*

"She found that true. So have I. Ah! . . . *creativity in destructive circumstance* . . . Now *there* is a miracle!

"God did not remove the unpleasant fact of my life.

"He enabled me to find creative use . . . *even now!"*

"The Redeemer God at work in unpleasant circumstance . . . now *there* is a miracle! I can only bow humbly, gratefully, worshipfully as tears erupt in the wonder."

The manuscript disappeared inside the publisher's house. My body toppled into extreme complications. My most constant activity was prayer. There was little strength for more.

And then the published book arrived at my door.

When I could sit up, I wrote this account to my brother.

"The day the book came, I was so weak I could hardly hold it. Finally I picked it up and it opened to the last page of the chapter on compression and I found there the haiku I had written long ago in ICU:

> Evening star wishes
> Never to come true and yet
> Butterflies on wing.

"Tears filled my eyes and my heart almost exploded as the impact hit me: EVENING STAR WISHES . . .

(All those myriad things I had planned for a lifetime)
Never . . . Never . . . Never . . . to come true . . . and yet
BUTTERFLIES ON WING!
Beauty . . . even now.
Joy . . . even now.
Wonder . . . even now.

"When Bill came home, I read the haiku and told him it best succinctly expressed my life-philosophy, even my theology. He held my hand, his eyes sooty with sympathy, his ears understanding the suffering threaded in my voice.

"Later we talked about haikus; how to write one; its three

major characteristics. I thought nothing of it since he always kindly shows an interest in things that intrigue me and are of no interest to him!

"He went away.

"Later in the afternoon, a dozen pink roses arrived from the florist. When I opened the card, to my incredulity, I found that he had taken time from his pressured schedule to figure out how to write haiku . . . and to write *two* for me on this momentous day. I would like to share that card with you.

> CONGRATULATIONS!
> *Winter's frigid blast*
> *Howling winds and snow; soon comes*
> *Bright Spring Harbinger.*
>
> *All tomes paper made*
> *Like fall leaves all decay while*
> *YOU are eternal.*
>
> *With all my love, Bill.*

"Again, my eyes filled; my heart bulged with emotion . . . but it wasn't caught on the first part of my haiku . . . ah no! I had moved to the second . . .

AND YET BUTTERFLIES ON WING!

"Even now . . . the love of a man so deep for his wife that he would learn how to write a haiku in celebration with, for even *of*! How beautiful!

"My life is limited inside four walls. And yet a steady stream of books, dramas, and musicals outreach, even around the world . . .

BUTTERFLIES ON WING!

"Of even greater beauty: Three men love me for the quiet, simple essence of me . . . even inside a fragile body where listening is often my greatest gift. These men cherish me in my small cocoon . . .

BUTTERFLIES ON WING!

"So here is the book. I hope its contents will bring you knowledge, challenge, perception of me, of my loves, *and* of my God. He *is* a Redeemer."

That book was written as a way of addressing the mystery with life.

That book was tangible proof that God wastes nothing when we give Him a chance to redeem. I had no thought, in the beginning, that its contents would ever be shared with more than the relative few who wrote personally to me. But in His time, in His way, He enabled me to find creative use . . . in unpleasant circumstance . . . even to the masses.

That book was proof of His promise: I will do miracles . . . I was "the bird with the broken wing" with a dream of being a Catskill eagle. Genie wrote: "She flies."

That book brought me the tangible articulate call to personal focus in the haiku, written long-ago and forgotten,

> *Evening star wishes*
> *Never to come true and yet*
> *Butterflies on Wing!*

20

You Might
Just Make It
After All!

When I came home from the Denver hospital with the full awareness of "limitations," Mary Tyler Moore had just completed her long-running series. Tributes and accolades were poured out by national media.

Our local television station responded by booking two Mary Tyler Moore reruns back-to-back every afternoon. I was, thus, able to spend an entire hour every day with this charming, warm actress.

When the show began its run, it was the story of Mary Richards, small town girl, leaving to try to "make it" in the big city. The opening of each show portrays her driving away, fear in her big brown eyes, and the underlining musical lyric concludes: "You might just make it after all."

Every afternoon, I would look forward to my "hour with Mary." And twice during that hour (at the beginning of each of the half-hour shows), I would bow my head and pray with all the earnest sincerity of my being: *Please, may I make it after all?*

"Making it," by that time, had reached such realistic levels that it had nothing to do with astonishing drama. I was praying, not for the great miracle, but for steady, plodding, day-after-week-after-month-after-year *redemption.*

Oh, there were times when I would look wistfully at others in our world who experienced all the definitions of dramatic miracles for which I prayed! And I would say: *O Father, all things are possible unto Thee. Why do You give to these . . . and not me?*

The answer was always the same. As He responded to Peter's query concerning His treatment of John, so He responded to me: "What is that to thee? Follow thou me."

And so I had to leave those healthy, successful, racing ones with the drama I yearned for . . . and walk this dark, lonely, painful road with God . . . *trusting Him.*

I wrote in my journal:

Oh, wow! How hard it is! Trusting Him. I don't see any point in what has happened; it doesn't make any sense; it doesn't equate justice on any scale I know.

Isn't it unfair?

Wouldn't it be best to do it my way?

But day after weary day . . . nothing happens . . . and I am left completely without 'miracles' as I want to define them.

So. I have to turn my inner eyes upon a new definition of the term and allow it to be His . . . not mine.

All things are possible unto Thee. I know that.

And in the light of that, I pray, as did Jesus, 'Let this cup pass from me" . . . A miracle by MY definition . . . PLEASE!

Yet not what I will but what thou wilt.

Oh! How excruciating are those words to form.

But I have. I do.

I look back over the past years of 'solitary confinement' and I find miracles dazzling and sizzling all through . . . not one of which had one thing to do with my definition.

But that they were true God-miracles, I cannot doubt.

An example: the hyperactive overachieving professional became the despised "little old lady" complete with ivy!

Don't fight a fact, Ruth.

Deal with it!

Twice daily, I earnestly prayed: *please may I make it after all!*

And "making it" was all wrapped up in the "little old lady." Oh! how I shrank from that image in ICU. I . . . I . . . I . . . *a little old lady!!!* It was intolerable. Unbearable. Completely unacceptable.

But gradually, carefully, slowly, hesitantly, I opened to "her." I began growing ivy for the first time in my life and rejoiced in its beauty. I spent hours at the window looking out at the purple majesty of the Rockies hulking into an azure sky. And . . . I made friends with television.

I not only found Mary Tyler Moore, but I found the "talk shows" where Dinah and Dick could "come to call, bringing their friends." I found the documentaries on PBS, the "classes" in everything from history (which I've always adored) to flower-arranging, the special news shows, William F. Buckley's *Firing Line*, Bill Moyers' *Journal*. I became involved in political shows and am probably the best informed voter in our country!

I tried to keep my mind active, busy, stimulated at all times. Loneliness is "the feeling of not being meaningfully related." Who said "a little old lady" could not still participate in life?

And gradually I learned to laugh about it.

One night, my three men were home. They were in the kitchen fixing the meal. I wanted to be with them, but was too weak to sit up. So I went in and lay on the floor in front of the refrigerator. Bill and Billy were teasing Ron about a girl and he was disclaiming interest. I said: "Ron, now I hear she is a very nice girl."

He said: "Oh, Moddy, that she is, but Daddy didn't marry you just because you were a nice girl!"

Bill had just taken something from the refrigerator. As he deftly stepped over my prostrate form, he said: "No, I married her because she is so vibrantly healthy!"

And we four laughed.

Laughed.

Now *there* is a miracle!

My doctor has been amazed at my finding the miracle of a change that he, and the others, had known was *impossible* humanly. He said: "There is a warm glow about you that I can bask in. You really did it: you found 'life-changing wisdom' to make you happy . . . even . . ."

He paused with his eyes twinkling.

I picked up his line.

"Even as a little old lady!" I concluded for him.

He laughed. "I didn't have the nerve to say it. But these last months, I have remembered the agony in the hospital when we talked about life-changing wisdom. How you rebelled at the boundaries! How you scorned becoming 'a little old lady!'"

Mischief danced in his eyes.

"I was writing my report in the medical records after your last visit and I almost wrote: 'She is a most wonderful little old lady!'"

We both laughed.

"Anyone reading that would think you were nuts!" I told him.

He grinned. "Not professional lingo, to be sure. But significantly meaningful. Its definition, you know, is 'Ruth really made it after all!'"

My eyes misted.

He didn't know.

By that time, the reruns on television had progressed to the point in the show where it was obvious Mary would "make it" in the big city. The last line of the opening lyric was changed: "You're gonna make it after all."

Now . . . I could bow my head in gratitude and sing along my version: "I'm gonna make it after all!"

Now *there* is a miracle!

I have learned to live within the "limited parameters." And God *has* redeemed.

I received a letter from a young businessman in our church. He said he had been at a men's prayer breakfast where the topic of unanswered prayer arose. That led to discussion of my illness. They talked of the night, two years before, when they had gone, with the rest of the congregation, to kneel about the front of the church in united prayer for the miracle of healing. They spoke of the confusion they felt when *nothing happened.*

And then they came to some surprising conclusions. This young man, who said he had never written a letter to anyone outside his family, was so impressed he felt he had to write to tell me of their decisions.

His letter was a beautiful gift and, when I responded to it, I wanted him to know *how* beautiful:

"I have lived through lonely day after weary month after painful year . . . with the unsolved questions . . . with the faith (the substance of things *hoped for*; the evidence of things *unseen*) . . . the mystery . . . and then came your letter. You said: 'I believe God has *used* your condition and honored you like no other person in the church.'

"Oh, Mike! I still can't read those words without tears. They mean too much. Don't you see? You are unequivocally asserting that the faith in the Redeemer God using even unpleasant circumstance for good is *vital, viable, at work* . . . even now.

"There are no words to describe the darkness, the human loneliness, the enshrouding incomprehensibility of all this . . . and yet I have determined to be open to redemptive use . . . I have prayed not to waste the illness. And now you write: 'I believe that the ministry from your home is as strong and meaningful as any ministry in the church.'

"The tears flood. I cannot stop them.

"Mike, if your report be true, we are, indeed, standing on holy ground. Because your letter says that, on the ground of senseless, destroying, wasteful illness . . . on *that* ground, the Redeemer God has enabled me to make *creative use.*"

But it is true.

In spite of "the book," in spite of Genie's assertion, in spite of Mike's letter, it is true.

Pain is still pain.

Suffering is still suffering.

A burned life-carousel is still my fact.

But in the life of Jesus and those who have followed/follow Him closely, we find Love refusing to despair over the world . . . we find Sharing refusing to isolate itself from pain and suffering . . . we find Companioning clasping human life with all its absurdity, grief, and sorrow.

As I study the life of Jesus . . . look at Francis of Assissi, Mother Teresa, I find that the degree that they *accepted* the suffering, to that same degree they offered their lives to alleviate human despair.

Jesus and His followers *love God in and through and beyond*
their own sufferings. They lash out neither at the pain nor the
God who allows it. They simply offer their lives to it, and love.
They address the mystery with life.

Prior to this illness, I loved God on the level of a myriad of
exciting careers and life-going-my-way. In the illness, I learned
to love God deeper down, farther back, and behind that. I have
even learned to love . . . and feel His love . . . without *words*.

That illumination came in a recent hospitalization.

Complications had arisen and immediate threat to my life
resulted. Bill was called at his office and he rushed to the hospital. He arrived in time to be a part of the storm of rushing in
machines, equipment, starting new IVs. When the crisis point
seemed to be past, at least for the moment, the doctors and
nurses tiptoed away.

As I became conscious, I saw him sitting in the chair beside
me. Through half-closed lids, I looked at his beloved features and
drew strength from his presence. Consciousness came and went
but, always, when I looked, Bill was sitting beside me.

As I began to revitalize, it occurred to me that this active,
articulate man had not spoken. For hours, he had sat in total
silence by my bed. I was intrigued with the reason.

And then suddenly it occurred to me: There are no words to
say. Bill understood the dangers, the pain, the imminent loss
. . . but he had no wisdom to erase the danger. He had no tonic
to dispel the pain. He had no antidote to prevent imminent loss.

There were no words.

In his eyes, I could see the tender, compassionate love en-
folding me. In the drawn muscles of his face, I could see the
anxiety and concern for me. But there were no words.

And suddenly I understood.

Perhaps it is when God is *most* tender with me that He is
most silent. He fully understands "the ground on which I stand"
and He is with me. And His Presence is in a dimension of
strength-giving that defies verbiage.

Bill had sat with me during these long hours without a word.
I could construe that to mean that he was not concerned with my
suffering. My knowledge of the man caused me to know better.

God had been with me during these long years with the most prolonged periods of silence I had ever known. I had construed that, many times, to mean that *He* was not concerned with my suffering. My knowledge of His Person should have caused me to know better.

I had wanted my prayers answered verbally, tangibly, dramatically. Nothing happened. Nothing was said.

And so, at times, I screamed in anger or cried in disappointment that God had withdrawn, leaving me alienated, alone.

I was wrong.

I could see it in the illustration of Bill setting beside me hour after hour in the hospital . . . and in a sudden flash, I could see it in the scene on Golgotha when Jesus Christ hung on a cross. The Father-God had *no words* to say.

Feeling the human anguish of loneliness and need for words, clues, answers, miracles, Jesus, too, had experienced alienation and cried in despair: *"My God! My God! Why hast Thou forsaken me?"* The Father-God was consumed with compassion, yearning sympathy, empathizing love . . . but there were *no words.*

Perhaps . . . When God is the most silent . . . He is the most concerned.

The thought was new to me.

I turned it over and over in my mind, examining it on all sides. I had equated answered prayer with words, miracles, drama. Now I was beginning to equate answered prayer also with silence, patient waiting, His Presence with.

Yes! That was what meant so much to me in that moment: Bill was *with* me. I was weak, suffering, needy . . . and he was *with* me. From his presence came his gift of love and strength. What was fact was fact. *Words* would change nothing. Only sharing could bring comfort.

That was true with God.

One of my friends sent me a motto: "The God I serve parted the Red Sea and made iron to swim. He will do the same for me."

I believe the first sentence. I am open to the second.

But I know that the Damascus Road experience only happened *once* to the great apostle Paul. All the rest of his life was lived in the dailiness of human life with a "thorn-in-the-flesh" ever-present. C. S. Lewis wrote:

> That God can and does, on occasions, modify the behavior of (natural law and free choice) and produce what we call miracles, is part of the Christian faith; but the very conception of a common, and therefore stable, world, demands that these occasions should be extremely rare.

At another point he wrote:

> . . . fixed laws, consequences unfolding by casual necessity, the whole natural order, are at once the limits within which their common life is confined and also the sole condition under which any such life is possible. Try to exclude the possibility of suffering which the order of nature and the existence of free wills involve, and you find that you have excluded life itself.

For many, as for me, suffering is the major stumbling block on the road to Christian faith. I now see that it is something basic and integral to human life, like sharps and flats are to music. Take away sharps and flats, and there is no music. Take suffering away and there is no life (except as robots in a paradise). The point is not to single out individual notes (such as my own personal tragedy or Kenna's divorce or Kay's baby's death or Burrell's paralyzing accident) and debate their *why's*.

The point is to focus on the *who* of the Redeemer God and bypass the *whys* and ask *how* can I participate in contributing melody to the whole composition. Sharps and flats are imperative in good music. So can the creative use of my individual pain if I am open to the Redeemer Composer.

Antony Powell called life "a dance to the music of time in which he who strains may hear secret harmonies." If one resists the truth of suffering, it can destroy the spirit. Such denial can be like a foreign malignant body that not only exists in the soul, insidious and irreducible, but it also exudes the suffocating carbon monoxide of defiance, ultimate despondency, and despair.

I remembered from childbirth that resisting pain only intensified it. Stiffening my body against the contractions of the uterus in its uncompromising will to deliver my sons made the suffering ruthless and relentless. My doctor had said over and over: "Give, Ruth. Push, Ruth. Work with the pain, Ruth."

Had I not been able to do that, a Caeserean section would have had to be performed. Had my body not agreed to the suffering of birth, it would have received a wound.

That seems analogous to life. Pain is inherent in human existences; to resist it creates another wound. There is an old saying: "Man is born in another's pain and perishes in his own." Suffering is a reality at the core of human life.

I read the Book of Job and it seems that his message was: "I will trust God in loss.

"I will trust Him in suffering.

"I will trust Him in grief.

"I will trust Him, yea, I will believe in Him in *every* circumstance of life.

"I will trust Him in life-debris . . . before life-carousels.

"I will trust Him . . . *'Though He slay me.'*"

To parallel Job, my creed would have to be:

"I will trust God in a quiet, lonely house.

"I will trust God in human pain.

"I will trust God in the death of all my dearest hopes.

"I will trust Him, yea, I will believe in Him in *every* circumstance of life.

"I will trust Him in life-debris . . . before burned lifecarousels.

To use my old book title, "I will trust Him . . . *no matter the weather!*"

But such affirmation still leaves suffering as the darkest and strangest of life's mysteries. It gives *no* answers, *no* clues, *no* solutions.

I almost memorized the Gospels which give the record of Jesus' suffering. He went into the wilderness forty days and forty nights but no maudlin details are given. Only short declarative sentences that do not arouse pity for the agonizing Christ. Through all succeeding accounts of His life, there is no attention given to the *why's* of the pains He experienced . . . only the succinct account of *how* He dealt with the realities He knew.

That became especially luminous to me on a morning when it seemed I had run out of answers to *how*. I had agreed to write a new play. But it seemed I had finally splattered into impossibility. I simply could not summon the strength to begin. And I knew if there was not the capability to write this play, there probably would be none for others.

The play was already in my head. The structure had been worked out in compression of time, characters, sets. My spirit was excited, challenged, but the body was sucked in an undertow of weakness that made it seem impossible to transfer the drama from brain to paper.

I had tried for days. I could not sit up for long. The swollen fingers would not move. The brain lay like a fly caught in syrup.

This particular morning, I lay in all my pea-green limpness, bypassed the *why*, and moved on to *how* the first scene could be best presented. At times like that, it is almost as if I try to lift the spirit out of the body, completely ignore its aches and pains, its limitations, and go on with work in the cerebellum.

As I focused with all energies I could summon on that opening, it happened! Like the coming of the sun from behind a cloud, the scene came full-fledged, full-fleshed. And in it was a character called Meryet, who was determined not to concede life as waste. She was a slave in Egypt. I was a slave inside a "limited" body.

As she came alive inside my head, I sat up. As I understood her spirit, the tears streamed down my cheeks. As I felt the surge of her courage, so I felt the in-marching of my own.

And as loudly as my strength would allow, I *shouted* in that empty house words that later became lines in the play:

Oh! I hate that word *slave!*
But I love the word *meryet!*
'Cause Meryet means courage and strength and joy
. . . And that's *just what I have!*
Courage to find my way out of this place . . .
Strength to *somehow* make my dreams come true . . .
Joy . . . it's gonna be mine . . . wherever I am . . .
Wherever I go . . .
No one's gonna keep me down . . .

In spite of all the bad things: the slave bond
        the suffering
        the impossibility of it all . . .
 In spite of all of that, I'm gonna have joy!

I got up then and went to the typewriter and wrote that entire first scene in the flush of the moment of my own determining to sing the lyric I wrote for Meryet:

I'm gonna laugh at every sun!
I'm gonna shout each step I run!
No matter if life is mean, I'm gonna find a way . . .

And there I left Meryet's song to make my own . . .

"No matter if life is mean, I'm gonna find a way to write this play . . . *even now!*"

I look back on that moment in my den and smile at the incongruous picture it must have been. Tiny weak lady squeaking out in little-more-than-a-whisper *her heart shout* that she refused defeat. Had anyone been peeking in the window, what a laugh they could have had.

But it was a pivotal moment for me.

I had been *giving* to the weakness. It was so easy to do that. Now after this sacred moment of my own personal victory, I wrote in my journal:

As I sat down to the typewriter, my heart was singing top volume as my fingers sped on the keys to record what was happening inside.
   I'm gonna laugh at every sun!
   I'm gonna shout each step I run!
I look now at that lyric and smile. Talk about incongruous. I smile for laughter. I whisper for shouting. I totter for running. But that is the body! That is only the body!
 Inside where Ruth lives . . . I am doing just exactly what I wrote:
 Laughing at every sun . . . shouting each step I run . . . determining: 'No matter if life is mean, I'm gonna find a way' . . . to write this play . . . and make it available for God-ministry.
 I don't know why I am so weak these days.
 I don't know why the fingers are so swollen and wooden.

I don't know why the brain so easily slides into molasses.
I don't know why . . . so, like Jesus, I'll by-pass it altogether and focus on how I may deal with what is.

And I did.
When later, I saw the play in printed form, when I received the Niagara of mail in response to its performances, I whispered in grateful worship of the Redeemer God: "I might just make it . . . after all!"

This, then, is what I can share with those whose "little boat" has entered the "dark fearful gulf" of a broken life.
This, then, is the lamp I can set ablaze to illuminate the shadowy course of others who may follow in the Journey of pain.
The knowledge of *who* bypasses *why* moves on to *how* which is the *holy ground* upon which the Redeemer God will enable you to make creative use of old-world debris . . . to build a new world.

This is His answer to our anguished cries.
And that answer changes the anguish of:

"My God, My God, *why* . . . ?"

to the hushed worship of:

"My God, My God . . .
You are Redeemer!"